# MY LIFE IN THE TWILIGHT ZONE

## Raising a child with autism

### By: Roberta Ruth Hill

# PREFACE

When I wrote this book, my intentions were to truthfully describe the events that unfolded within my life. I particularly wanted to show how abuse, chronic illnesses and Autism or any other disabilities can affect families, as well as the individuals that are experiencing these difficulties. In my attempt to explain all the events that transpired, I forgot to mention how I have been able to forgive any transgressions towards me or any personal mistakes that I had made during that period of my life. I hold no one liable for any negative actions towards me or my son, and I have been able to accept every experience, whether it is negative or positive as a learning tool for my own life. Please do not judge me or anyone in this book that made mistakes and take these experiences that have been written as a learning tool for your own lives. I realize that I did vent some anger or bitterness issues that were holding me down emotionally, but this was done more in an attempt to release these negative events from my life in a pure therapeutic way. The truth of the matter is that I wouldn't change anything that occurred within my life, because all these things made me who I am today and have made me stronger. Although, I realize now, that in telling of all these events truthfully and in a straight forward manner, that I failed to mention how forgiveness played a major role in my life.

My intentions in writing this book is not to hurt anyone, but to truthfully show how these events affected me. I hope that this book can help other people that have endured these same kinds of experiences, and that they can learn from my many mistakes. I just wanted for others to understand what it is like to go through these kinds of difficulties, and to educate people about Autism, abuse and Diabetes.

When I first told my son that I was going to write this book I asked him if it would be okay with him and he said "yes", but that he didn't want me to mention his name. I've written this whole book keeping in mind his wishes and so I kept his name anonymous.

## Acknowledgments

I would like to thank God, the Holy Spirit, Christ and the Angels for teaching me and patiently waiting for me to learn the lessons that I need to acquire on my journey in this life. Thank you for your constant support and love.

I would also like to thank my mother, Stella Forinash, for encouraging me to write this book.

# THE BIRTH OF MY SON

I was about to experience an event that would change the rest of my life forever, and I was very afraid of the way it was all unfolding very rapidly. It all began one May morning at work, when I began to feel an unusual sensation in my abdomen. Now, I was 23 years old and I was going through my first and only pregnancy, which was a new experience for me. I didn't really know what to expect with the labor pains and I still had about two months to go, so I didn't even realize that this is what labor pains are like in the beginning.

Hours later this unusual sensation turned into pure pain, and then suddenly I was very aware that I was in labor. My husband rushed me to the local hospital, and the team of nurses and the doctor monitored my condition. I laid on the gurney and tried to get through every contraction without yelling, which is what I really wanted to do. I thought of every kooky movie scene or television scene that showed women in labor, and suddenly I knew exactly why those women were always yelling, hitting people and telling off their husbands. It's funny how I always thought they were making child birth way more dramatic and outrageous, just so they could get lots of laughs. Well, it really is just like that, and I was marveling at the realism of it all, but don't worry, even though I thought about it, I didn't hit or yell at anyone.

My dad and my father-in-law came into the emergency room, and I can still remember a part of their conversation. I was hooked up to a fetal monitor, which

4

showed my contractions. They were very interested in this contraption, and were watching and discussing about each one of my labor pains as they would appear on the monitor screen. They would look at the screen and proclaim that I must be having a contraction, while I was going through a labor pain. It would have probably been funny to me if I wasn't going through the most intense pain of my life. I looked at them calmly discussing about this machine, and I just wanted to tell them something that I thought, but never did speak, so here is my chance to finally say what I was thinking on that day.

"Hey guys, remember me, the person that is hooked up to this funny looking contraption.....yeah, that person. I am experiencing the most intense pain right now, and all you two can do is look in amazement at this monitor. It really is annoying to hear you talking about each one of my labor pains and quite frankly, I just want to take a hammer to that thing." That monitor for all its high tech and graphics, was upstaging my labor pains.

Yeah, so much for an inspirational thought or recognition of an elegant and well thought out epiphany that would change my life forever. Well, if you were going through the most excruciating pain of your life, what would you be thinking about?

It was nice when my mom got there to visit me, because I knew she would know exactly how I felt at that moment. Women are always united in their shared experiences and there is always this unspoken truth between them.

Anyway, so the doctor decides to give me some medicine that is supposed to stop the labor, but it never really did, it just slowed down my labor pains. Thanks for that doc!

So basically, instead of having my son be born right then and there, I had to go through 3 days of labor and a tour of 3 different hospitals, before I finally achieved victory.

I never do anything in an ordinary way, you see, in my life, anything that can and may go wrong, usually happens to me. Yeah, I'm one of those kinds of people. You know the one that everyone talks about behind their back because of their unfortunate and unusual circumstances. Yep, that's me.

The hospital staff decided that since my labor wasn't coming to an end, that they should send me to another hospital that could deal with the complexities of a premature birth. They ended up sending me from New Smyrna Beach to Daytona Beach, in a very posh looking limousine with cool flashing lights and lots of cool technological gadgets. Oh yeah, did I forget to mention that I was very high at this point, and couldn't see clearly because I was experiencing double vision.

Anyway, so here I was going to Daytona Beach in an ambulance, and trying not to panic over what the paramedic had just told me. She said something like this, "I can deliver a baby, if I have to." I couldn't ever figure out if she was talking to me or if she was trying to psych herself up for having to deliver a baby in the ambulance. Fortunately, though, I did not have a baby in the ambulance, and I was very glad about that going right. After all, I still had some touring of the local hospitals and some traveling to do, before that was going to happen.

Many people come to Daytona to go to the world's most famous beach, or to attend the car races, and of course the college students and motorcycle enthusiasts come to party. Well, I had two of those covered, I was high on drugs and I was racing down the highway, but it was hardly a fun and exciting trip for me to take.

Just as they were pushing the gurney into the emergency room, I started shaking uncontrollably and couldn't stop myself. The nurse informed me that this was a side effect of the medicine that they were giving me. Personally, I think I was trying to dance, while I was looking at the psychedelic illusions of seeing two of everything, but who knows, it could have been a side effect.

After my lengthy stay of about one day and one night in Daytona Beach, I was informed that the hospital didn't have the right facilities for dealing with premature births, and so they gave me the choice of two different hospitals. Finally, I got to choose which destination I was off to next. Let's see, Gainesville or Orlando? Of course, I chose what every person on vacation or in premature labor choose, I chose Mickey Mouse land. I just hoped that Goofy wasn't going to be there to deliver the baby.

Again, I was chauffeured to another destination down the interstate, with my own personal mini bar included, and I had a cocktail IV in my hand. Ahh, I was living the good life. Fortunately, I was no longer feeling the labor pains, or any kind of weird side effects, and at this point I was feeling pretty darn good. I was just waiting to see where this adventure was going to lead me to next. Disney world would have been a nice place to give birth, and my son could have got an early start on amusement parks.

Well, the hospital where we arrived was called the Arnold Palmer Hospital, and it was the closest thing to

Disney that I had ever seen. They had a mini life size model of the Cinderella castle that is in the middle of Disney world, and they had paintings of Disney characters all over the walls. This place seemed more like a magical fairy land than a hospital, and I was impressed with everything there.

I guess my son finally decided that this was the place that the birth was going to happen, and I couldn't have been any happier to finally get the whole thing over with and done. My son can sure pick the best place in the world to make his entrance on Earth. What could be better than the theme park capital of the world? It's the most fun place to be.

I can still remember how crazy some things got there. It was a Mickey Mouse land, indeed. It seems like with that new medication, I was becoming more like a hippy, and just couldn't get enough of telling everyone how much I loved them. I was just really feeling good for a while there, but then I discovered that there was a side effect with this one, too. My mouth started to get dry so quickly, and I always felt like I had been sucking on cotton. They were not allowing me to eat or drink, so I was getting everything from my cocktail of IV meds, vitamins and fluids. It's a very bad feeling to want to gulp down a giant glass of soda, only to be given a small cup of ice to suck on instead. My lips became chapped and very dry, and I kept trying to moisten them but to no avail. I felt exhausted and this 3 day excursion into the unknown was really starting to get me down. In addition to all of this, my husband decided that this was a good time to start complaining about my family. I was already worried about our baby, and then he would talk to me about subjects that would      worry me even more.

I should have told him that he could walk out that door if he didn't want to put up with my family, but I didn't. Remember, I was still going through the hippy love and peace thing, so it was fortunate for my husband, that I didn't get mad. Although, I wasn't exempt from all of his anger issues, he was exempt from mine, because I was still deeply medicated.

I looked more like a robotic machine than a person at this point. I had a fetal monitor going around my abdomen, a pulse monitor on my finger, an IV in my wrist, and a catheter tube running up my leg. Every time I wanted to turn over, I would have to adjust all of these wires and tubes that were hooked up to me and it was just so annoying.

The pulse monitor reminded me of ET's red finger, because of the little red light on the end of the clothes pin like device. I felt like ET at that moment, except I didn't just want to phone home for help, but I wanted to go home immediately. Also, there were many monitors around me that would beep and hum at various times throughout the day, and it almost felt like I was a Borg on Star Trek, I was hooked up to a collective of machines and they told about everything going on with my body to the others. Okay, so I guess by now, you have figured out that I am a big sci-fi geek, but I still had to include these analogies.

I have since looked at the video that my family had taken, and I looked like I was stoned, with my unkempt hair looking similar to Einstein's hair. Basically I looked like the bride of Frankenstein, and even that might be too flattering. It was real freaky to look at myself on that video; I couldn't believe how bad I looked. Well, I had been so drugged up, that I thought that my hair was perfect and that I resembled a pillar of strength and calmness. Oh well, there goes that illusion, and I thought I had managed to look like a model through that whole thing.

Finally, the big day arrived; I was dilated and ready to give birth. The nurse told me that I could now start pushing, but I was in so much pain that this was the last thing that I would have ever wanted to do. I mean really, when you have all this pain, you just want to sit there real still until it all passes. But no way, that's when they tell you that you have got some work to do. So here I am in a position that I don't ever want to be in, with my private's open for all to see, and I have someone yelling at me to start pushing. Well, I yelled back, "I'm not going to push!" I really don't know how I thought I was going to get out of all of this stuff, but if there had been a way to avoid all of this stuff I would have tried. However, it's not like I had a choice in the matter. Of course, the nurse yells back at me and tells me that I am going to start pushing and I'm going to start with the next contraction. She gave me such a harsh look and I was so terrified of that nurse that I did just what I was told to do. If she had not got tough with me, I probably would have held out for awhile longer, so it was lucky for me that she spoke up to me.

I was in the main delivery room for about 10 minutes, and I was coughing all through out the pushing. Cough and push and cough and push, until finally my son had made it all the way out into this world. They ended up doing x-rays on my lungs after my son was born, and they found out that I had a touch of pneumonia.

On May 26, 1990, my son was born, and he was a very handsome looking baby. I can still remember how alert he was and the way he kept looking around at everybody. I had always heard that babies were kind of blind when they are first born, but my son seemed to be looking around and taking it all in and he seemed actually interested in everything in this world.

Once the nurse, put him into my arms, though, he seemed to calm down and went right off to sleep peacefully. I marveled over his tiny hands and feet, and loved how he looked in his cute little crocheted cap on his head. He almost looked like a tiny baby doll to me.

Throughout that whole wacky process, I learned a great many things about myself and others. I learned that God and my family are the source of my greatest strengths in my times of hardships, and without their support, I could never get through the tough times in this life. During this whole process, I was visited by my parents, my father-in-law, my cousins, my Aunts, my sister, my husband's friends and my grandmother. It was a comfort to have them all there for my son and I, which is something that I will never forget.

I also learned, unfortunately, that my spouse was not capable of giving me the love and support that I so desperately needed, but it actually took me another 14 months of his erratic behavior to realize that I didn't have to put up with his coldness and abuse anymore.

When I first became pregnant, I was so afraid and didn't know if I would be able to get through the pregnancy and then be able to raise a child. After the pain of labor was gone, and I held my son in my arms, I knew that I could get through any problem, great or small, or go through any pain for my child. I knew that I could do anything for him. He gave me a strength and courage that I didn't even know that I had, and that strength came from our love. That love started way before I even saw him or held him, like the egg that grew inside of me into a fetus and then into a baby, my love had been growing for him throughout that whole time, too. I didn't realize that in addition to giving birth to my son that I was also giving birth to a greater love than I had ever known at that point in my life. My selfish ways was transformed, as I became a mother that day, and that meant that I would learn to give more than I would receive.

They always say that when you marry your spouse that you become as one, but they never say that about becoming a parent. It seems to me though, that we also become as one with our children, as well. It is evident in the way that we care and protect our children; we treat them as if they were ourselves. Their pain becomes our pain, their joy becomes our joy, and their achievements become our achievements and through it all our love grows stronger and stronger.

Looking back, I realize that this whole experience was a preparation of what was to come. You see, the labor pains never really do stop, they continue in other less traumatic ways. The waves of emotions that come in the middle of the night, when you awaken with worry about your child, or the intense waves of emotions that flare up, when your child has argued with you and you don't know why they are so upset. The pains of all our labor to raise our child, continues to follow in cessation from one moment to the next. A world where parents are continually racing back and forth to put out their children's fires and to save their child from the dangers of this world is much like the roller coaster ride that begins with those labor pains

THE NEWS-JOURNAL

DAYTONA BEACH, FLORIDA
Monday, May 28, 1990

B

# Tiny lives are coaxed to healthy growth in neonatal care units

**By WILLIAM D.A. HILL**

Tiny lives surrounded the corner this week, babies in neonatal care units from that beautiful old hospital on the hill, Halifax Medical Center, to the ultramodern Arnold Palmer Hospital for Children and Women in Orlando.

Little ████████ Hill was supposed to arrive in July, but last week when my daughter-in-law announced a stretching sensation in her abdomen, the thought arose in my mind we might be heading for a premature delivery. We were. Brian's struggle began at Fish Memorial Hospital in New Smyrna Beach, where a generous and loving group of professionals explained in lay terms the risks to a 3-pound baby.

Late last Wednesday, the doctor sent the expectant mother and father to Halifax, where neonatal care was more appropriate to the needs of a 3-pounder.

Going to Halifax is like going to grandmother's house, a sensitive, warm place that always has the feel of home. From Cheryl at the front desk to the doctors, nurses and technicians in the Family Birth Center, we were met by skilled professionals with a warm, human touch. Through the nervous night spent at HMC, our questions were answered directly and candidly, and always with encouragement.

Thursday morning, an evaluation of ████ premature state and expected low birth weight led the doctors to order a transfer to Orlando's Arnold Palmer Hospital.

## IN THIS CORNER

Stella Mercer, my daughter-in-law's mother, joined me for a final conference with HMC's Dr. Lisa Gonsalves, who used plain English to tell us why the transfer was necessary and what to expect. Her parting words remain in my mind and in my heart. "The baby's chances will be good. Believe that," she said.

Arnold Palmer Hospital is part of Orlando Regional Medical Center, a sprawling complex of buildings that seems to grow by the hour. The Palmer Hospital opened last September, and is one of only four hospitals in the country — the only one in the Southeast — specializing in high-risk neonatal care. The hospital proudly points to a 90 percent survival rate among high-risk babies.

Palmer looks and is highest tech. Its people bring skills and abilities that seem like elements out of science fiction. Even the architecture is pure science. You expect to see eggheads in white coats here, and you do. But they speak to you!

In the blue-and-white sterile atmosphere of the second floor where the neonatal intensive care and preemie units are located, eggheads with personalities scheme to save the lives of babies born in crisis. They do speak a scientific style of English, but we found if you gently prod these noble intellectuals, they will get down to plain

SEE **CORNER**/ 2B

13

# □ **Corner**

CONTINUED FROM 1B

talk. It was in this futuristic place that ▆▆▆ was born.

On Saturday afternoon, many crises behind us, Brian, weighing three pounds and 13 ounces, cuddled in his grandad's arms for the first time. Tensions and fears for his life diminished, and his little lungs produced volumes of air. ▆▆▆ lips moved and his voice chirped as his old grandad softly hummed and sang "All through the night" while seated in a rocker in the special care nursery. In isolets and beds surrounding us, premature babies struggled to live.

A mother and father wearing sterile yellow gowns walked to an incubator near us and paused, looked. My heart went out to them because in that moment as I held ▆▆▆, I knew that mother and father longed to cradle their own child in their arms.

I can never forget when my son and his wife, tears creeping down their faces, held ▆▆▆ for the first time. Because of the medical scientists in that wonderful hospital, soon, maybe real soon, that anxious couple will hold their baby.

Among the direst neonatal cases with respiratory membrane afflictions like ▆▆▆, Palmer has a 70 percent to 80 percent success rate, said Dr. Gregor Alexander, director of the neonatal intensive care unit.

He attributes the success to adaptation of the Extra Corporeal Membrane Oxygenation (ECMO) technique to babies, and Palmer is the only place in Florida using it on babies.

How long ▆▆▆ will remain at Palmer can't be answered now. He's fought off his major crisis, and maybe he will be bedding in his mom's room on Memorial Day.

14

# THE MARRIAGE

The next four years were some of the most difficult times of my life. I was about to experience every kind of problem that can be tossed at a person. When I think back on this period of my life, it is very easy for me to compare my life to Job's tribulation period in the Bible. During this time period, I moved 8 times, endured some abuse, got a divorce, went through a custody trial, my son's onset of diabetes started, dealt with my son having seizures, went through a SSI trial, dealt with terrible tantrums and found out my son was autistic. In addition to all of this, I lost my good credit, had family members turn against me and was unable to work.

I wish I could say that I was making all this stuff up, so that my life would look more dramatic, but all this really happened to me. If you had to label my life's story for a book or a movie, you would have trouble figuring out whether to label it as a drama or a comedy.

During my son's first two weeks of life, he spent a vacation at Orlando, Florida, in a very posh resort with servants to attend to his every need and whim. They called this place the Neonatal Intensive Care unit. My husband and I separated during some of this time, and so we visited our son separately. I visited every day, and I was able to hold him and to feed him. He was such an amazingly tiny baby, but he had such a huge personality, that his body couldn't seem to contain it all. He seemed much older and wiser than a premature baby should. Now that I am looking back, it seems to me that my son has a very old soul, and that shined through in a countenance that just glowed. During the 18 years that I have had the privilege of knowing him, I have watched him endure so many tragic things and yet there is a joy of life that he displays so often. He has been amazing to watch all of these years.

Getting back to my story, my husband and I worked things out, and after two weeks, we took our precious son home. Apparently, after a premature baby reaches his goal weight, they evict him from the resort, I mean hospital. So my son went from Orlando to New Smyrna Beach during his first few weeks of life, of course, he had to experience the beach on his vacation to this new world. We were living with my husband's father at the time, and were about a half mile away from the ocean. Not a bad place for my son to come home to after his time spent in Orlando, and we enjoyed having him home with us.

At some point, we ended up moving to an apartment in Jacksonville, Florida, and my husband had got a job as a marine mechanic, which didn't last long. You see my husband was one of these guys that thought jobs were like a revolving door; he kept entering them and exiting them in very brief periods of time. He revolved through so many jobs when we were married, that even I got confused as to where he was working half the time. We didn't stay at the apartment long, before he convinced me to use a credit card in my name that I had received in the mail, as a down payment on a mobile home he had found for sale. Oh yes, it was the American dream, to own a place of our own, paid for in my credit. So, of course, I jumped at the chance of having our own place, but I forgot to read the fine print of the nonexistent contract

16

between my husband and me. You know the invisible contract that says, if he decides to stop making the payments, that I am held liable. Yeah, I was a total moron on this decision, wasn't I?

By this time, he had changed jobs again, and was working for the cable company. We had moved into our new home, and for a short while, I was actually happy, until reality started rearing its ugly head again. He stopped making the payments on the mobile home, and I was getting really depressed. He sold cable, so his paycheck reflected that with his commissions. One paycheck would be really good, and the next one would be really bad. He controlled all of our finances, so I never knew where all the money was going, until I got an overdue bill in the mail. I don't know why he stopped paying for our mobile home, but his decision led to ruining my credit.

Some idiotic and frightening stuff happened at this home, which I will never be able to forget, no matter how much I want to forget about it all. One time I can remember, I was enjoying reading a magazine, while my son was taking his nap. My husband came in and took the magazine from me and ran out, I ran after him and saw him run outside and throw the magazine in the car and lock it up. The only thing that I could think to do was to lock the front door, which was a big mistake, because he grabbed an axe and started to hit the door. I unlocked the door immediately and ran for my bedroom. Looking back, that wasn't the smartest thing to do, when I let him in there with an axe in his hand, but at the time, I was afraid that he was going to destroy the door and the mobile home with that thing. I thought I could get back to my bedroom and lock the door, but he was much faster than me. He followed me into the bedroom. He threw a decorative metal tin mailbox at me and I ducked just in time to avoid being hit. I've heard of airmail before, but this was ridiculous. It hit a frosted decorative glass window that went in between our bedroom and the bathroom, and the whole glass shattered everywhere. Even now as I am writing about this, the whole thing still doesn't make much sense to me. I still don't know why he did that and I have to wonder if maybe he was on drugs or maybe he was just mentally unstable. It was one of the more bizarre moments of my life, where I had wondered if I had turned down some dark road into the twilight zone.

Another incident that happened involved me making the worst mistake of my life. We were having another argument, which seemed to happen quite frequently with him, when I decided to take some Tylenol pills in front of him. I just swallowed a bunch of the pills. I don't know if I was trying to kill myself, or if I was just trying to show him how miserable I was. It was a huge mistake, and I really regret that I did that. As you can see, neither one of us, was actually mentally stable by this point. Our marriage was so bad, and I was under so much stress that I was clearly becoming a nervous wreck at this point.

I don't know how all of this could have affected our baby, but it's not hard to see how emotionally distraught we were, and how that could have had a detrimental effect on our son. I know that our son had to be feeling the tension that was in his home. It was a bad environment for a baby to be living with all that stress within his home. I have always wondered if that might have affected him in some negative way. I hope not.

My husband convinced me to go to Charlotte in North Carolina to try to find a job. We did, and he found another job at a cable company. We sold so much of our stuff at a yard sale, just so we would have enough money to move. I can remember selling stuff that I cherished, but we had to do that to have money. I had to always make sacrifices in that marriage, he had sold my car when we were living at the apartment, my credit was ruined and now my stuff was being sold for this move. We owed so much money on our mobile home, that we knew it was only a matter of time before we would get thrown out.

We moved into an apartment in Charlotte, and it wasn't the best place in the world. I can still remember hearing the sirens of police cars all the time while we were there. It was a very bad neighborhood, and not the kind of place that you want for your child to be.

At some point we rented a mobile home, my husband changed jobs again and was working as a security guard. He also started to volunteer at a local fire department. It was at this time, that I actually had more time to myself, and I was able to think about my marriage. I started calling my family more, and read a book about abuse that my mom and a friend picked out for me.

One night we had another argument, and he ended up holding me down on the floor. At some point, I ran into the bathroom and locked myself inside. He got the door open with a knife and when I saw him coming in through the door, I snapped. I started hitting him repeatedly. He ran out and went over to the neighbors to call the police. Ironically, after all his abuse towards me, when I finally decided to fight back, he ran like the coward he was and told everything to the police. When I think of all the times that I could have called the police on him, but I didn't, it seemed like some sick joke had been played on me. The police came and questioned both of us. They asked me if I wanted to press charges, but I did not. It wasn't long after this event that our marriage finally came to an end.

I was in pain for a few weeks after he had held me down on the floor, and every time I got up or sat down, a pain would shoot through my chest area. I never went to the doctor, so I don't know what he had done to me, but I was sore for quite awhile.

He left me and our son, and went back to Florida. He took everything of any material value, but left his most valued treasure behind.....his son. We were left behind in a mobile home, where the rent was past due, as well as other bills, like the electric and phone. He left us with no money, but promised that he would pay child support. I would like to say that he kept that promise, but of course, he never intended to pay child support for his son. Our son was just 14 months old at this time, and he would grow up without a father.

So there you go, that was the extent of our marriage, and it was one heck of a roller coaster ride. There were plenty of twists and turns and ups and downs along the way. It was exciting and dangerous at the same time, with fear and confusion as to what would happen next, but finally this ride had to come to an end.

It was a fireworks show from the beginning and to the end, but this wasn't to be the finale to all the explosions of our marriage. In order for fireworks explosions to be seen at their best, they have to happen in the darkness of the night. Later on, I was to find out that my husband had some more firecrackers to explode on his way out. He did not go off quietly into the night, without first setting off some more fireworks during my darkest of night.

\*\*\*\*\*\*\*\*\*\*\*\*\*\*\*\*\*\*\*\*\*\*\*\*\*\*\*\*\*\*\*\*\*\*\*\*\*\*\*\*\*\*\*

## LIFE'S STRUGGLES

My life really changed when I married Dave,

I'll always remember the way he would behave.

I found out four months after we married,

about a secret that he alone had carried.

He had been calling on the phone his ex-girlfriend,

and did this behind my back, which I reprehend.

I found out about his child from a stranger on the phone,

that he kept a secret, which I couldn't condone.

I found out that I didn't know who I was married to,

and that I had made a big mistake when I said "I do".

I was the only one working at the time,

and he wasn't contributing even a dime.

He was going to school to get a better job,

but all I heard were complaints with a sob.

He twisted my leg when I was pregnant,

and I slowly began to feel          disenchant.

21

Some days he would get mad and break some things,

and I had trouble coping with all of his mood swings.

I was in my seventh month when I started in labor,

but what I will never forget was my husband's behavior.

A problem erupted between my family and Dave,

and while I was in labor I would have to listen to him rave.

He would come into my room just to complain,

and he didn't seem to worry about me being in pain.

I went through three days of labor, which was hell,

and then I would have to hear him yell.

I was worried about weather my baby would be OK,

and to God I would find a peaceful time to pray.

He was born healthy in the month of May,

and I will always remember that wonderful day.

He was so alert on the first day of his life,

amid all the turmoil and all the strife.

His body was small and he had very tiny feet,

and had a look about him that was very sweet.

The same day that he was born, they did an x-ray,

and I found out I had Pneumonia that very same day.

The next day Dave came into my hospital room to yell,

and the nurse threw him out of the room, which was swell.

We decided at the time to separate,

and the first time in months I felt great.

I wish that I would not have gone back to him,

because when we got back together everything turned grim.

We moved away and Dave became in control of me,

and because I was so busy taking care of a baby I couldn't see.

He sold my car, which left me dependent on Dave,

and then ruined my excellent credit which I forgave.

Then he moved me to NC after selling stuff for the move,

and I followed whatever he said even if I didn't approve.

During our whole marriage he would go from one job to another,

while I stayed at home trying to be a good mother.

There were sporadic incidents of abuse,

and he did some things to me that I can't excuse.

When he was fourteen months old, we had a fight,

and he threatened to take our son, which caused me to fright.

He ended up leaving our son and me all alone,

with no money, car, or a home; which I can't condone.

He promised that he would pay child support,

but paying a couple times was really short.

He came up with every kind of excuse,

and I think he thought up every story he could use.

We had to move in with my mom and dad,

which really made me look so bad.

I had no means to help me get back on my feet,

with Dave leaving me with nothing left me with defeat.

How could I get a job with no car or childcare?

the only thing I could do is go on welfare.

Dave really stuck me good,

How can you live with no money for food?

It's hard to live without money, a car, a home, or without credit,

especially when caring for a baby and when you have a debit.

He left with an unpaid electric bill that was in my name,

and he put me into a situation, which caused me shame.

Then he called up many members of my family spreading lies,

and many members of my family starting gossiping like flies.

My dad's mom said that we should not live with my mom and dad,

when I heard about that it really made me feel sad.

I had everything taken away from me in such a short time,

and I was down on my luck and was broke without a dime.

I was looking for a job when my son starting getting sick,

then he seemed to get sicker really quick.

The hospital found out that he was a Diabetic Type one,

and they told me that diabetes was genetically prone.

I had to learn about the diet, shots, and blood test,

and there was so much information, it was hard to digest.

Our son was in the hospital for about six days,

but in that time we learned all about the diabetic's ways.

A few months later I told Dave about what our son had,

and he blamed me for the diabetes, which made me mad.

He started having seizures in the middle of the night,

we would all wake up to a sound that caused such fright.

At some point I learned that Dave got a divorce from me,

now I knew that I was going to be finally free.

But he also got custody of our son, which I couldn't believe,

and he got custody through his lies to deceive.

I sent papers to the judge to show proof of the lies he told,

and the judge removed the custody clause, which was bold.

I started custody proceedings in NC and informed him,

the chances of him getting custody were pretty slim.

I got custody of our son without telling lies to Dave's surprise, because honesty is the best policy say the wise.

We went to Celebration Station to celebrate,

and we had a fun time and felt really great.

But our problems weren't exactly over just yet,

because he started having violent outburst when upset.

I had him evaluated and found out he was delayed,

and when I learned that I was somewhat dismayed.

He was diagnosed with autism when he was four years old,

and none of us knew what else would unfold.

There have been years of problems within the schools,

and many teachers have treated my son and me like fools.

Well, now finally things are going really great,

but I know that hell will have to freeze over before I will want to date.

\*\*\*\*\*\*\*\*\*\*\*\*\*\*\*\*\*\*\*\*\*\*\*\*\*\*\*\*\*\*\*\*\*\*\*\*\*\*\*

# DIABETES AND SEIZURES

The fairy tale endings of marrying a handsome prince and then moving to a castle and living happily ever after, seemed more like some comedy that Hollywood had dreamed up, than the cold harsh realities of true life. When I think of all those young girls that grow up believing in the fairy tales in books and movies, I think that they have been told a lie that will screw them up for the rest of their lives. It was a fairy tale that told them that they could kiss a frog and make him into their prince, but they never tell you that you can kiss a prince and he can end up turning into a frog. Sadly, the fairy tale never did begin and was never going to be a reality in my life, because life isn't a fairy tale, and that's a cold hard fact.

I had no where to go, but either a homeless shelter or to move back in with my parents. I had no car, nothing of real value, overdue bills, bad credit, no home and a baby that relied on me. This is what my husband left me and our son with and he seemly didn't care that he provided nothing for his child to live on after he left. Prior to our marriage, I had my own car, a good job, and excellent credit, so I can't believe how low I had sunk in less than just two years time.

Despite all of the difficulties of our reality, I was actually happy at this time. It was a huge weight lifted off of my shoulders, and I felt free. I had been the loneliest in my life with that man, than I have ever been before or since. There is nothing worse than having someone in your life, but still feeling all alone in the world. That was how I had come to feel in that marriage, like I was all alone, but with a husband. I should have been getting the love and support that I needed, especially with being a new mom, but instead I got put down a lot.

Looking back, it was a huge mistake to marry that man, and I will never fully understand why I made that decision. I had been warned by a friend to not marry him, but I think I was so lonely, that I convinced myself that being with him was much better than being alone. In reality though, I would have been much happier if I had just stayed alone.

I had to decide whether to stay in a homeless shelter on cots and with a bunch of strangers, or go live with my mom and dad for awhile until I was able to get back on my feet again. Of course, we ended up moving in with my parents, and I was grateful to be staying with them, although I would have rather had my own place. I wasn't particularly thrilled with having to move in with them, but at the time I didn't know what else to do.

We moved into an apartment at first, and then into a mobile home that my parents had bought. I applied for welfare, Medicaid and food stamps, which is something that I thought I would never do, but real life has other plans. Both my parents worked at that time, so I couldn't look for a job, because I didn't have access to a car. We were living in the country with no public transportation system to rely upon, so I really needed a car desperately.

At this time, I just tried to look after my son, and tried to be the best mom that I could be. I started getting my son caught up on all his vaccinations and health needs, as well as doing other things to prepare him for a daycare. I had been trying to potty train him, but it wasn't working out. He was urinating too much, to even keep him in dry underwear.

After my mom quit her job a few months later, I started using her car to look for a job. I started filling out applications during my son's nap time, while my mom watched him. It had been about six months since my husband had left, and I was still unable to get back on my feet. There was no child support, so I needed a job badly. I finally had found a job at a factory in Asheboro, but sadly enough I was never able to go to work for them, because everything changed again.

Just about five months after my husband left, I noticed my son was starting to get sick a lot, and so I took him to the doctor. The doctor thought that my son had a virus and an ear infection, and so he was being treated with antibiotics, but I noticed that he kept getting worse. We took him to the hospital at Asheboro to get him checked out. I told the doctor that he was drinking a lot and urinating frequently. His response to that was to tell me something that made me feel so stupid. He said, "Well what goes in must come out." I thought, "Duh, I didn't know that doc thanks for telling me that pearl of wisdom." I ended up leaving with the feeling that I had wasted my time by going there for help. Well it ended up that the symptoms that I told him that day are classic symptoms of diabetes, so that doctor was the ignorant one for ignoring what I had to say. He never checked my son's blood sugar level, which could have saved him from going through a very traumatic experience.

One morning I went into my son's room to wake him up, and instead of seeing my son, I saw another face staring back at me. His eyes were sunken inside his sockets, and I was aware that he had lost more weight. His whole countenance had changed, and it frightened me so much. He had been vomiting everyday, and he wasn't getting any better on his medicine. I very quickly called the doctor's office and told them that I needed an appointment as soon as possible. I told them that something was very wrong, and my son wasn't getting any better, instead he was getting worse. They told me to bring him in immediately. Once the nurse saw him, she couldn't believe how different he looked after only a few days since she last saw him. She checked his vital signs and the next thing I knew, she was calling for an ambulance.

We were in the ambulance and heading for the hospital, when the EMT checked his vital signs. The next thing I knew the sirens got turned on and the ambulance driver increased the speed. I started praying immediately, because I knew that something was really wrong. My mom was following the ambulance and she later told me that she was praying, too.

We got to the hospital and the staff was checking out my son. They kept asking me the same questions over and over again, and they were focusing on the two bruises that he had on his head. I kept trying to tell them all of his symptoms, but I feel like they were more concerned about the bruises. Again, I felt like I was being ignored, and that frustrated me, since I was only trying to get some help for my son. It didn't take long to put it together that they were evaluating me for signs of possible abuse and neglect. I told them about how he was walking around the house like he was drunk, and he kept falling. He had got two bruises on his head from falling on the coffee table, and I thought that the dizziness was because of the ear infection. My mom came in at one point and she told them everything that I had been telling them, and she had brought pictures with her to show them how he looked before he got so sick. I think that was when they started to focus more on his symptoms after they realized that my mom had observed all the same things that I had. Looking back, I realize just how bad everything looked, and he did look like he was an abuse victim. If he had died, I would have been charged with abuse and neglect, and would have been sent to prison probably, but luckily they took a blood sample.

We knew he was diabetic, when we overheard a nurse say to put him on an insulin drip. He was so confused and hyper, and he kept going back and forth between me and his grandma, and he did this for hours. They finally admitted him to the hospital and they took him up to the pediatric floor. When we got off the elevator, everyone just stared at us, and it was the weirdest feeling. My son was placed in an ICU unit that was right beside of the nurse's station.

We didn't understand why everyone was just staring so closely at us that first day. We thought that maybe they still suspected abuse, but that wasn't the reason for their curiosity. Later on, we found out why everyone was so interested in my son. A nurse told us a few days later that my son's blood sugar was extremely high and that it was 1,103. The staff had been told to prepare for him to come up, but after learning the details, they didn't expect him to make it to their floor. They thought that he was going to die. They had a patient a few weeks before that had a blood sugar at that level and her brain swelled and she went into a coma and died. When the nurse told us about the girl that had died, for the first time, I realized how close he was to death. He had survived and we had seen another miracle. My son was a miracle twice now, he had survived a premature birth and now he had survived the onset of diabetes. What are the odds of a baby surviving so many complications? My son is truly a gift from God, and he is living proof that God can work miracles anytime that he desires.

During the week that my son stayed in the hospital, I had to learn how to give shots, all about the diabetic diet and how to test for ketones and his blood sugar. It was so overwhelming for me, but I tried to learn all that I could. I gave my first shot to a nurse that was training me. After training on oranges, she wanted me to experience what it was like to give a shot to a real person. I was nervous, but I was able to do it properly, and I was just thrilled that I was able to do the shot at all.

After a week, my son was released from the hospital and we were very happy to have him come home. One day though, soon after he came home, I had a meltdown and I guess the pressure of dealing with the schedule of diabetes really got to me. I told my mom that I didn't want to do shots anymore, and I basically had a little fit about having to deal with the diabetes. It's not like there could be anything done about it and I knew it wasn't all just going to go away like a bad dream, but I still had to freak out for a moment. I just needed to vent some steam and cry about the injustice of it all. Although it was more like a volcano going off then steam being vented, I just let out all of this emotion that was pent up inside of me. My mom snapped me out of it, like only a mom could.

She said something to me that shocked me back to reality. She said something like this, "If you don't do the shots, then your son is going to die." That snapped me out of it pretty good, it wasn't like I had a choice in the matter and I realized that there was no way I could get out of doing the shots. I ended up doing shots for about 14 years, after thinking I couldn't possibly do it at all. In life, we get used to doing things that we think at first is impossible for us to do, and that is just how life can be sometimes.

During his hospital stay, it took a team of nurses to hold him down for each and every shot, because he fought against them so strongly. When he came home, this did not change and I required the help from my parents to hold him down while I did every shot. I became so reliant on their help at that time, because I knew that I couldn't hold him down and concentrate on doing the shot at the same time. He was just too strong for one person to do it all by themselves. It was like he had a super strength to him and I never quite understood how he could fight so forcefully and be so small. However over time, once he got used to the routine, I was eventually able to do the shots without requiring the assistance to hold him down and that made it easier.

One night we woke up to the most unpleasant sound that I have ever heard in my life. I checked on my son and he was having a seizure, and we didn't know what to do. If I remember right, I checked his blood sugar and found out it was low. I started to give him something sweet in between his convulsions, and after a few minutes his seizure stopped. We informed his doctor and she made an insulin change, and later on my son went to see a neurologist for some more tests to rule out any kind of a seizure disorder. We found out that some diabetics are prone to seizures with a low blood sugar episode.

It is the most heartbreaking thing to watch your child have a seizure. No words can even begin to convey the emotions that sweep through your mind, when you experience seeing someone you love shake and jerk uncontrollably. His seizures got worse throughout the years as he got older, but also became less frequent. He becomes unconscious when he has them now, but back then his eyes stayed open during the entire seizure, and his eyes always looked glassy and dilated when he had them back then. That peculiar sound he made as a small child always alerted us to any problem at night and it was like having an alarm going off. I know that if he didn't make that sound during the night, he would have died, because I would have never been able to help him. That was another miracle to have that sound to alert us to any problem during the night.

At some point, I decided that I needed to tell his father about the diabetes, even if he wasn't apart of his son's life anymore. He wrote a nasty letter back to me accusing me of lying and then he also said that if he did have diabetes that I had caused it from neglect and because I had been giving him the wrong diet. He was never supportive as a husband, so of course he wasn't going to be a supportive ex-husband either. He never came to see his son, or never offered any kind words to help us through our difficult period, but that's the kind of father that he was going to be for the rest of our son's childhood.

I was supposed to go to my job, when my son was in the hospital, but I never showed up or even called them to let them know what happened. I was so distraught with everything, and I stayed with my son during his entire stay in the hospital and learned all that I needed to know to take care of him. After he came home, we called some daycares and found out that none of them could give shots and blood glucose test, so I stayed home and cared for him myself.

It had been about six months since my husband had left, and I still didn't have a car or child support and was not back on my feet again. Everything was looking dim for the future, and I thought that this was about as low as things could get, but sadly, I was wrong. I still went through much more than I ever could have even imagined, because the nightmare continued.

\*\*\*\*\*\*\*\*\*\*\*\*\*\*\*\*\*\*\*\*\*\*\*\*\*\*\*\*\*\*\*\*\*\*\*\*\*\*\*\*\*\*\*\*\*\*\*\*

## Diabetes

**My son got diabetes when he was eighteen months old,**

**And it was a vicious disease the way that it would unfold.**

**He had frequent urination and was thirsty throughout the day,**

**And then it got worse with vomiting that didn't go away.**

**He didn't look like my son, when I woke him up one morn,**

**And his weight loss and sunken eyes seemed to forewarn.**

**The ambulance took him to the hospital and I began to pray,**

And at the hospital he was diagnosed with diabetes on that day.

That was about eight years ago when our lives did change,

And now we struggle to keep his blood glucose in a normal range.

He has to have three shots and many blood test per day,

And has to limit exercise whenever he does go out and play.

He limits his sugar, fruits and carbohydrates at his meals,

And let's me know what his blood glucose is by the way he feels.

I get tired of having to give shots that hurt when they stick,

And his fingers are so scarred up from all the finger pricks.

I have had to deal with insulin reactions that were very severe,

And seizures in the middle of the night is what I always fear.

High blood sugar is what I fix with an insulin shot,

And when sugar is low, he gets his candy that I allot.

My son and I are hoping for scientist to find a cure,

To put an end to this disease, that so many have to endure.

And when that day comes we will all celebrate,

About a terrible illness that the scientist did eliminate.

\*\*\*\*\*\*\*\*\*\*\*\*\*\*\*\*\*\*\*\*\*\*\*\*\*\*\*\*\*\*\*\*\*\*\*\*\*\*\*\*\*\*\*\*

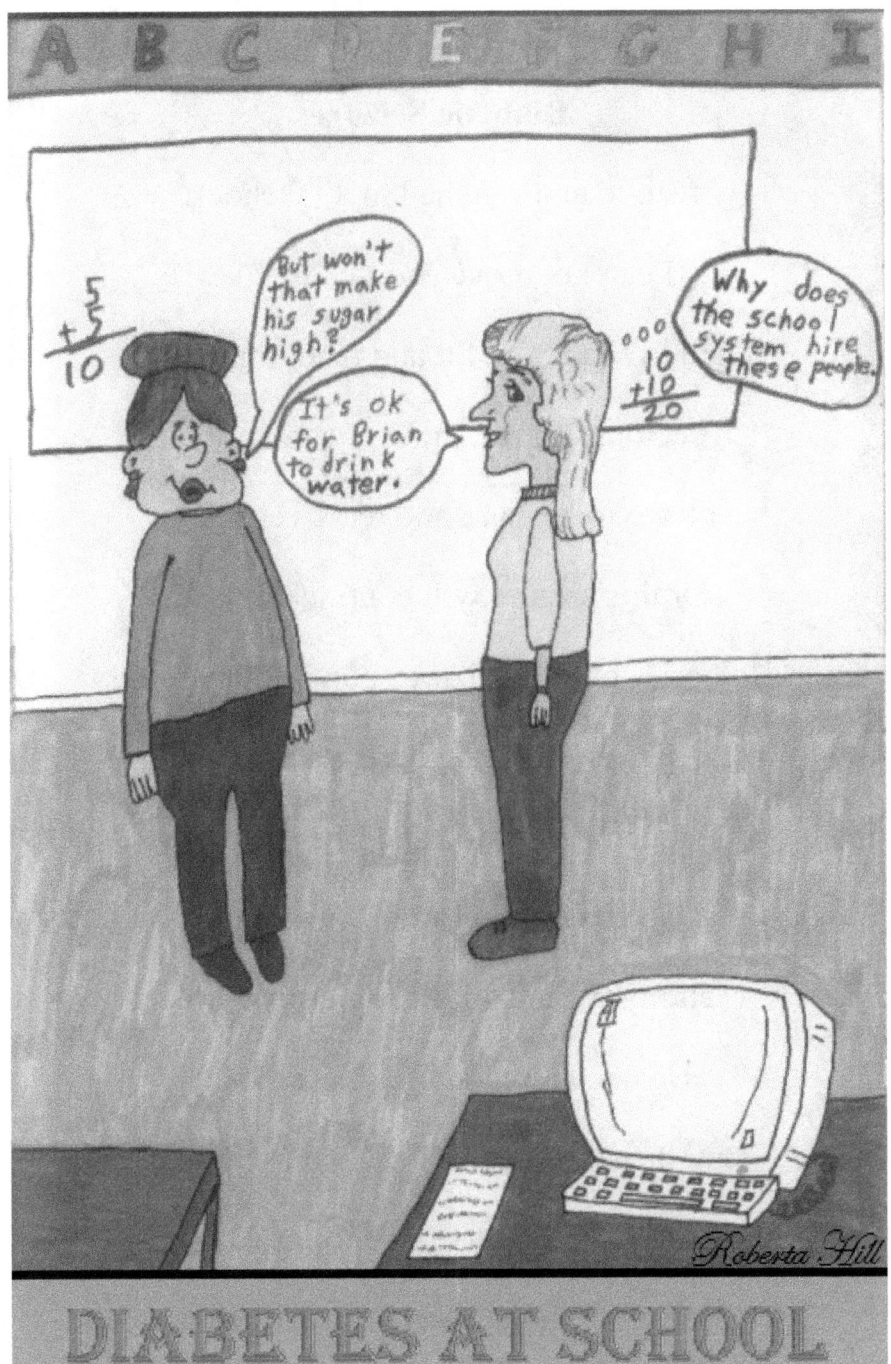

\*\*\*\*\*\*\*\*\*\*\*\*\*\*\*\*\*\*\*\*\*\*\*\*\*\*\*\*\*\*\*\*\*\*\*\*\*\*\*\*\*\*\*\*\*\*\*\*\*\*

## Diabetic Seizure

I stood and watched in total shock,

I can not move and I can't talk.

I had to snap out of it and react right now,

Precious time of shock, I can't allow.

I have to be calm and react very fast,

Or this seizure will continue to last.

Memories of past seizures pop into my mind,

Is there anything sweet that I can find?

I feel helpless inside and I begin to pray,

God, please help my son to stay.

I tell my parents to get something sweet,

He needs something sweet to eat.

But, he goes unconscious and I feel fear,

This hasn't happened for about four years.

I give him honey and hope he wakes,

The seizure ends and he no longer shakes.

My parents called for 911 on the phone,

I'm glad that we are not all alone.

He wakes up suddenly and tries to eat,

But he resist the honey that taste so sweet.

He is confused and still unaware,

I hold him in my arms and just stare.

My beautiful son is still alive,

And will continue to grow and strive.

My son is the most enthusiastic person I know,

None of his many battles in life ever show.

I'm amazed at my son's resiliency to bounce back,

And I hope he never has a seizure attack.

\*\*\*\*\*\*\*\*\*\*\*\*\*\*\*\*\*\*\*\*\*\*\*\*\*\*\*\*\*\*\*\*\*\*\*\*\*\*\*\*\*\*\*\*\*

**A Slave To It**

With four times a day,

Prick and stick is the way.

Needles are all around me,

That's what I hate to see.

I can't get away from it,

Because I can't quit.

A schedule that is cruel,

A schedule for a fool.

Life was once carefree,

It made a slave out of me.

I hate it when I give a shot,

I feel like a villain somewhat.

A pin cushion of skin,

Shooting the drug within.

A job I never asked for,

Trapped in a sugar war.

Can these chains unlock,

Promises race against the clock.

Will there be a cure today,

Or will the slavery continue to stay?

These shackles and chains do hurt,

There are complications to divert.

I'm tired of being just a slave,

Stuck with the schedule       diabetes gave.

# THE CUSTODY TRIAL

At some point during this time period, I learned about some devious things that my ex-husband was doing to me behind my back, which seemed like some kind of sick revenge against me. He started calling many of my relatives to complain about me and my parents. Wasn't that so considerate of him? He is so lucky that I didn't start calling all his friends and relatives, but fortunate for him, I am not the kind of person that does those kinds of things. He called my two grandmothers and some of my uncles and aunts. It was embarrassing to me and I felt like he did this to cause some divisions between me and my family.

My paternal grandmother that was complaining about me moving in with my parents was the only one that talked to him for awhile. I kind of saw this as being a betrayal to me, and my relationship with her never recovered. I needed a grandmother that would stand up for me and not one that would complain about me or listen to my ex-husband's lies.

I finally managed at some point to hire an attorney through Legal Aid, so that I could get a divorce. It was at this time that I received some more shocks that added further emotional suffering on top of everything else that I had endured.

I found out that my ex-husband had already got a divorce in Florida and had somehow sleazily got custody of our son. It was a total shock to me, and I couldn't believe that he had managed to pull that deception off so easily. He had already taken so much from me and now he wanted to take my son away from me, too. At any point during this time, he could have kidnapped his son away from me and I would have not been able to do anything, because the law would have been on his side. It was a very good thing that I told him about his diabetes, because otherwise he would have snatched him away from me at some point. I think that was the only reason why he didn't take him away from me.

I sent out for the divorce papers and found out all of the nasty details of the divorce and custody trial, that I was neither invited to attend or even given the courtesy of being told about the custody. He had made out like I left him in Florida and he left out all the details about us even living in North Carolina. Therefore Florida had jurisdiction over the custody trial, even though it should have been our son's home state. I sent all kinds of papers to prove that he was living in North Carolina and to show that he left us and that it wasn't the other way around. Fortunately I had all kinds of papers that he failed to take with him when he left. After all the television, stereo and the surround sound system were all important items for him to take, but his papers weren't valuable enough. Ironically, the stuff that he took with him was also bought with my credit, which, of course, he didn't pay it off either. He had managed to leave behind my most valuable asset to getting custody, but that never would have happened without my mom. I almost threw out all of those worthless papers before we left, but my mom managed to convince me to keep those papers that I considered to be trash. It was another miracle perhaps that I kept all that stuff, and that he left his trash, because it wasn't worth any cash. In the long run, those papers were the most valuable thing he left me, because they helped prove that the state of North Carolina had jurisdiction over the custody case. Up to this point, I never knew that trash could be worth so much to me, but this trash was more valuable then all the treasures I had ever had.

I sent some of his speeding tickets with his North Carolina driver's license number and some of his check stubs and Id's for his many different jobs that he had when he lived here. Oh yes, I sent proof of every word that I wrote to the judge, so that he would know that I wasn't lying, like my ex-husband had done. Jesus said, "That the truth shall set you free," and you know what, for me and my son, it did.

Oh yeah, I forgot the best part of his devious little plan. He had me set up to pay the child support. You know, the child support that he wasn't paying for his son, was now something that he was trying to get from me. Wasn't that so nice of him? It is moments like this that I know, demons do exist and sometimes they are in the physical form. How had he managed to sell all my stuff, sell my car, ruin my credit, take everything of value and get custody of our son? I couldn't even begin to imagine how evil that man was in everything that he did towards me.

It is for this reason, that for the last 21 years of my life, I have managed to stay single. Loneliness is much better than the betrayal of a loved one, any time. I have paid for my mistake of ever being with that man in so many ways throughout the years, that I can't even think of anything more torturous than what all he did to me. I paid for that relationship in the fear and tears of abuse that continued long after he left.

In the custody papers, I found out that my name had been forever soiled by him in a legal document in the court house for all to see. He told so many lies about me that it was almost laughable, if it had not been so painful to read. He basically made me out to be the most awful person, and it was so vengeful and cruel. That was his final act of abuse, and what he said has always haunted me to this very day. The damage that he was able to do to me in such a short amount of time, has forever changed me and the person that I used to be will never be found again. It is because of him, that I can't seem to trust people and I find it easier to just hide myself away from the world. I have so much emotional damage that I can't seem to function in the way that everyone else does.

Getting back to what happened, the judge in Florida struck the custody clause from the divorce papers, and so my attorney got to work on setting the court date for the trial in North Carolina. I started getting my paper work together, and asked my son's doctor if she could write a letter on my behalf for the custody trial. She agreed and wrote a letter about my son's diabetes which stated that I was capable of taking care of him. She also wrote that it would be detrimental to have him taken away from my care.

I also had my son's diabetic nurse as a witness at the trial. She had been so supportive towards my son and I during his hospital stay and we remained friends with her for a few years. She always seemed like a grandmother to me, and I was grateful to have her as a witness to testify about how I was as a mother.

The court case was swift and I got full custody by the time it was all over. Unfortunately, although he had managed to get an order for me to pay child support to him, I wasn't as lucky. He was able to slither his way out of all that because he was unemployed at the time, and he got away with not paying child support for 12 more years. When he finally did have to pay years later, after the state pursued him vigorously, he kept paying it on and off and his payments were never a reliable source of income.

The Judge was very nice and he put in a clause to help protect my son, which I was very pleased to have in the custody papers. My ex-husband was required by the law to get some training about diabetic care and then he had to submit proof to the court before he was even allowed to have visitations with his son. He never got the training so that he would have his visitations and I never understood why he didn't find it important enough to do this for his son.

I even let that snake of an ex-husband actually see his son after the trial, even though he wasn't supporting him or had not visited him after he became diabetic. We had actually found one day care that agreed to watch my son during the trial. I thought that if they were able to do a good job with taking care of him that now maybe I could finally get a job. When we got back to the daycare, I saw my son acting rather strangely and no one was attending to him, so after we left the building I tested his blood sugar. My ex-husband was so shocked and he actually had a look of pain, when he saw me prick our son's small finger and squeeze out some blood onto the test strip. If I remember right, his blood sugar was in the 30's, and so I got him a snack very quickly to try to bring it up, so that he wouldn't go into a seizure. That was the first time he stayed in that daycare and the last time, because I realized that only I could take care of him. His father's visit was very short, because he was anxious to get back to Florida, and I was glad when he left.

After all that was over, I decided that it was time to get my son tested by some experts, because we were all aware that something wasn't quite right. Just before he became diabetic, we all had noticed some unusual things with his behavior. Like when we tried to call his name, he seemed to ignore us. At first, I thought he had a hearing problem, but after getting him tested I found out that his hearing was very good. There were other strange behaviors, too, like not making eye contact for long, never sitting down and his speech wasn't where it should be for his age.

My son started to have these really horrible tantrums, and many times he would trash his room in a fit of rage. There was a few times that his bedroom door would be hard to open due to the fact that he threw so much stuff around his room that it would all block the door. It was kind of scary at the time, because I feared that I might not be able to get into the room, but luckily every time I managed to force the door open. I didn't really know how to deal with these explosive burst of rage, and so I asked my parents for help. They both tried to help me and were as perplexed as I was when they were unable to control his behavior, as well. It was a sobering reality, when I realized that he wasn't having the normal tantrums that come with a typical toddler.

After having him tested, I found out that he was really delayed in a lot of things in his life, and they diagnosed him with a Pervasive Developmental Disorder. It was recommended that I get him into a program where he could get some help. He started going to a place called the Enrichment Center, which was for preschool children that had developmental disabilities. He went for a few hours a day and they taught him many different skills and gave him speech therapy.

During this time, it gave me the opportunity to do some more things. My mom suggested that I should apply for disability, since I was unable to work because I had to take care of my son. I did eventually apply for SSI, which I felt would help us get back on our feet again. After initially getting turned down, we went to an attorney to help us fight for the disability. After about a year, he was approved and we got about a years worth of back pay. It was at this time, approximately 1 and1/2 years after my husband left, that I finally got a car again. Finally everything was starting to turn around for us, and we were starting to get back on our feet again.

We looked for a used mobile home and found a nice one with three bedrooms that we bought. All of the back pay didn't cover the entire balance, so I had to take the rest of the money from my parent's credit card and I started making payments to them each month. It was worth it, though, and I was excited to be moving out finally.

Our new home was wonderful, and I really enjoyed being able to be on my own again. My son really loved our home, too, and I could tell he was as excited as I was about our move.

Now that we had our own place again and I finally had a car, I was able to explore more options that I hadn't even considered before. I was able to enroll my son into a school program for head start. He went there for about six hours a day and he got his speech therapy. I was able to apply to a community college, and to start taking some classes. It was so wonderful to be able to go back to college again, and I started taking courses to prepare me for the nursing program.

# AUTISM

My son was going to the head start program, and I was beginning to see some progress with his language development. I started going to college and at some point I chose to take a CNA course to get certified as a nursing assistant. It was actually kind of fun and was very easy, so after I did my clinical and took the final exam I had my license for being a CNA. This gave me something to do while I was waiting to enter into the nursing program.

He had a very nice teacher, and she really started to help me with some new ideas for potty training, which was something that I had been struggling with immensely. Ultimately, it seems like rewarding his successes by giving out stickers was the one thing that worked very well. Even though I had been praising anytime he would use the potty, I believe he needed something to visually see, rather than just hearing the words. Apparently with autism, it wasn't enough of an incentive to make their life easier or to feel more comfortable without the wet diapers; they need colorful stickers or some kind of tangible reward to make it worth the effort. He was potty trained very quickly using that method, and I was surprised that it actually worked. He was three years old when he became potty trained completely, and I was so thrilled.

My son had all kinds of peculiar ways during this time period of his life. I can remember he use to collect rocks. How is that weird you might ask? Well every time we were in the parking lot of his school, which was filled in with ordinary granite rocks, he would pick up a hand full. He kept putting the rocks in the car and I always had to keep cleaning them out all the time. I guess you could say that everyday he rocked and rolled back home. That was his normal everyday routine, to collect some rocks from the parking lot everyday he went to school. If I had not kept throwing them back onto the parking lot, well I guess we could have made a parking lot of our own after awhile.

Back then, my son had the ability to memorize words from movies, commercials and from other people. It was not uncommon for him to repeat a line from a movie at anytime. This is called echolalia in the autism universe, and it means that they will repeat what others say word for word. I always saw this behavior as more of strength, because if he was able to memorize words, then I knew he would be able to learn anything. Of course though, there were times that echolalia could really get on my nerves, and many times I felt like there was a parrot in the room repeating what I had just said.

Another interesting thing that developed into a routine was his constant need to always have stuff with him where ever we went. This was apart of him since he was a very young baby, and I can remember him always crawling or walking around with objects in his hands. It was so commonplace when he was a baby, that my sister nicknamed him as "no hands baby", because he always had his hands full. If we ever went to visit his grandparents, then it was absolutely imperative that he had to have all kinds of objects and toys with him at all times. Over the years all of his various collections was stuffed into many grocery bags, so that he could manage to carry it all with him to every location that he was going to visit. I can remember thinking about how my son's behavior resembled the homeless people or bag ladies that travel around with their bags and grocery carts filled with lots of stuff. I kind of have to wonder if some of the homeless people might have mild autism, but were never actually diagnosed, because they were just considered to be eccentric or just a little bit unusual. It was something that became kind of embarrassing to me, because it was so weird. I hated having to explain to relatives or other people about why he did these things. Although many attempts through the years were made to break this habit, nothing ever actually completely worked and he still has a need to have stuff with him to this very day, even though he is now 22 years old.

The teacher kept hinting around about the "A" word, and I kept finding it more and more difficult to ignore that word. To me, autism was that guy that Dustin Hoffman played in "Rain Man", and I just wasn't ready to accept that yet. So, it was more comfortable for me to keep making excuses for his bizarre behavior then to accept fate, and boy did I have some interesting reasons for why he did all of this stuff. Maybe it's because he doesn't have another sibling to show him how to do things, or because he doesn't have a father around him, or, you know, it could be because of the diabetes. Another one of my favorite excuses, had to do with the fact that he was a preemie and they are always delayed because they were born too early, but subtracting two months from his actual age still didn't seem to account for all the weird stuff he did. Anyway, you get the idea, I'm sure every parent of an autistic child, tries to explain everything in an intellectual and precise way, but eventually you succumb to the same question. Why the heck is my son acting so weird?

Eventually, I did clue into the teacher's constant hinting around about this or that behavior being autistic like, even though, I had thought that I did a pretty good job of trying to ignore this whole thing. I decided to lookup some information about autism, and what do you know, it pretty much consistently described his behaviors over and over again. But there was at least one ray of hope for me; it also described things that my son had never done. So one day I marched into my son's school with a list in my hand of the things that he did that were like autism and the things that he didn't do, and was convinced that perhaps he could still get out of this label being placed upon him.

When he was four, fate kept knocking at our door. The teacher wanted for me to get him tested by a team of professionals, and was going to set up an appointment for him. Of course, I knew that none of these behaviors were going away and that he needed special help, so I consented to have him tested by TEACCH, which was an organization which diagnoses and helps children with autism. There were many different people that evaluated him that day and tested him for his overall cognitive level of functioning. It was decided by this team that he was best described as having mild autism, and that later on there could be other diagnoses added, such as mental retardation.

Well, that first day I was alright with his diagnoses, but for some reason the next day it just sort of hit me very hard and like a ton of bricks. I realized that there was no going back to my old ways of thinking. I couldn't just think or say, that he was going to catch up or that everything would just turn around someday soon. There was no more hope left for a brighter future, and I knew that these bizarre behaviors weren't just going to go away like I had hoped that they would. It was my day of reckoning, and I had to find it in me to just accept that this is the way that things are and nothing was going to change.

When a parent has their child diagnosed with autism, they go through the grieving process. You go through the anger phase, and the questions of "why me" or "why my child" seem to pop into your head quite consistently. It isn't like you love your child any less, but it is like you have to realize that your child may not be able to accomplish all the things that you were hoping that they would be able to do and experience. That is why you almost go through a grieving process, you have to let go of all your own perceptions and expectations for your child, and you have to realize that your child might not achieve all the things that you expect from them. It is a really scary time, and I'm sure many parents do get quite depressed during this adjustment period. Then after you finally come to an acceptance of your child's situation, you can move on with your life and adjust to everything accordingly. I can remember that this was a very difficult time for me, but basically I just hung in there until I didn't feel angry or bitter anymore.

The period of time when you are going through this acceptance process is emotionally compounded by the fact that you have to deal with the most unusual circumstances on a day to day basis. You almost have to begin to accept that your life is in no way ever going to be normal again and you get so used to different types of behavior that you no longer see it as abnormal for your child. This makes the way for some interesting looks, stares and comments that you will get from teachers, family and any onlookers along the course of your life. Everyone will point out all the unusual things that your child does and look to you for an explanation, but what they don't realize is that you're so used to the weird behaviors that it has become normal to you. It's like trying to explain everything that is mysterious in the universe; you just can't do it because it is impossible to understand, so you just eventually accept that and move on.

Although in the beginning, I frequently found reasons to explain my child's unusual behavior. Like the tantrums, for instance, becomes a survival tactic that has kept him alive all these years. I can remember saying things like, "well, it sure is good that he is such a fighter in life, and I bet that is why he has survived his being a preemie, his onset of diabetes and all the seizures." I found the successes in everything I could, like a miner hacks away through the rock and dirt to find the gems; I meticulously looked for my child's strengths among all the bizarre behavior.

I started saying or thinking, the oddest things that I never noticed before then. "Yeah, so what if he likes to carry tons of stuff in his pockets. I hardly use all my pockets, so at least he is using everything he has with him." Everything becomes a new and unique way of looking at the world, through your child's eyes. I actually started to see some brilliance in the autistic perspective, and no longer disregarded every routine as being totally useless.

Suddenly, my son's need to collect granite rocks became a rock collection, and so I went with the flow. Well you know, if you can't beat him then join him. Through the years, I managed to take that routine and get him interested in different kinds of rocks, instead of just grey and dull looking granite rocks. I started taking him gem mining and gold panning, so that he could see that there were so many different varieties of rocks than granite. That routine ended up being an interesting hobby that we have both enjoyed over the years together. He started that hobby and I jumped in and got involved with it, too, and it brought us closer together.

The diagnoses of autism is not an end all to hope of ever living a regular life, it is just the start of a new beginning or journey that you will undertake. In this new autistic universe, you will undoubtedly see many new strange and exotic things that you can't explain, but upon observance you will always find a new perspective that you never realized before. I have learned so much from my child that it could probably fill volumes of knowledge, and I think most parents would agree with that statement.

None of this is to say that it isn't hard, because the truth is that it is a very hard journey to have embarked upon in my life, but I am just trying to say that it is worth the experience. Along the way young parents will discover so many new things about life that will outweigh all the trouble and heartache that you will undoubtedly experience.

Right now there is an epidemic going on that seems to be growing bigger and bigger by proportion every single year, and that is one reason why I wanted to write this book. I want to let all the young parents know, that they will survive this and they are going to learn so much and grow as a Human being. It is not as devastating as you might think it will be, but that you will get many pleasant surprises along the way that will delight you and enrich your life so much.

When my son was first diagnosed there was 1 in every 10,000 children that had autism, but according to the latest statistics it is now 1 in every 88 children. That is such a big increase that I can't even begin to wrap my head around the changes that have occurred in the last decade.

Many of these children will experience the same symptoms that my son has, and although I can't offer you a solution to every problem, I can reassure every parent that everything will turn out just fine eventually. You just have to adjust and move on and never try to look back at what could be, but look at what is precious before you now.

\*\*\*\*\*\*\*\*\*\*\*\*\*\*\*\*\*\*\*\*\*\*\*\*\*\*\*\*\*\*\*\*\*\*\*\*\*\*\*\*\*\*\*\*

## Autism

He didn't look at me when I was talking to him,

And the chance of getting his attention was very slim.

Those were some of the problems when he was 1 year old,

And I didn't know what would through the years unfold.

I wanted to believe that everything was alright,

That he was normal and his future was bright.

During these days he started to get sick so fast,

But I thought that this sickness would soon be in the past.

Diabetes Type 1, I thought could be to blame,

For why he was so hyper and didn't respond to his name.

Was diabetes causing him to act this way?

I wondered if this strange behavior would stay.

Because he was delayed, I put him in a special daycare,

I still didn't realize he had autism and was not aware.

He started having violent tantrums at the age of two,

And it left me feeling helpless, not knowing what to do.

He would lose control and trash his room in a fit,

And some days were so bad I just wanted to quit.

It was always scary when we went to shop,

With all the tantrums in the store I would have to stop.

We got mean looks and stares from people where ever we went,

And I began to ignore these ignorant people that I came to resent.

He was diagnosed with mild autism at the age of four,

And I had a hard time accepting it and tried to ignore.

I thought he could be cured and tried many different things,

But nothing would cure the autism or the behavior that it brings.

I have been hit, bit, kicked and scratched for many years,

And his destructive behavior has left me with many fears.

There were times when I thought about giving up the fight,

But I held in there for my son which I believe was right.

There were many behavior problems within the schools,

Because he didn't understand how to follow all the rules.

It took forever to teach him how to safely cross the roads,

And it took years to learn how to deal with violent episodes.

His communication skills and speech are more normal now,

From all the years of work at school and home which showed him how.

Many different teachers and speech therapist have helped him,

And without their help the future might have looked grim.

I have seen through the years, many autistic traits go away,

But there are still a few traits that still seem to stay.

I am finally starting to see the progress of many years,

Those years of work that was filled with many tears.

Today my son is outgoing and he is a very intelligent boy,

And every time I look at him, I am filled with so much joy.

He has taught me more about life, then I ever could have learned alone,

Watching him overcome obstacles and deal with health problems on his own.

I use to think that it was only a parent's job to teach the kid,

But now I know, with my sons help, better than I once did.

\*\*\*\*\*\*\*\*\*\*\*\*\*\*\*\*\*\*\*\*\*\*\*\*\*\*\*\*\*\*\*\*\*\*\*\*\*\*\*\*\*\*\*\*

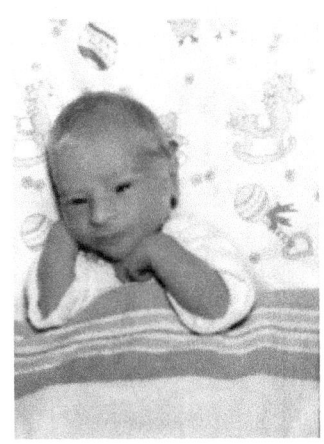

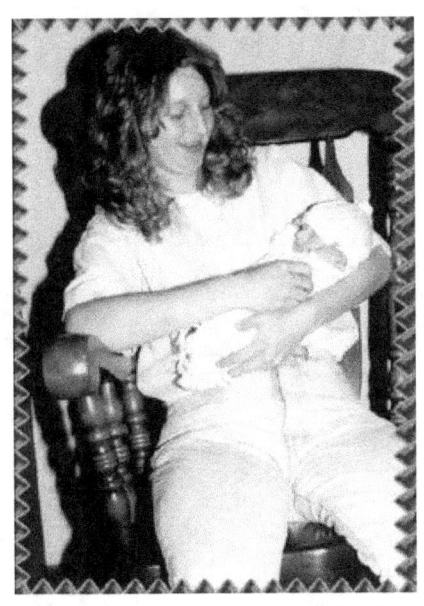

MY SON 1990

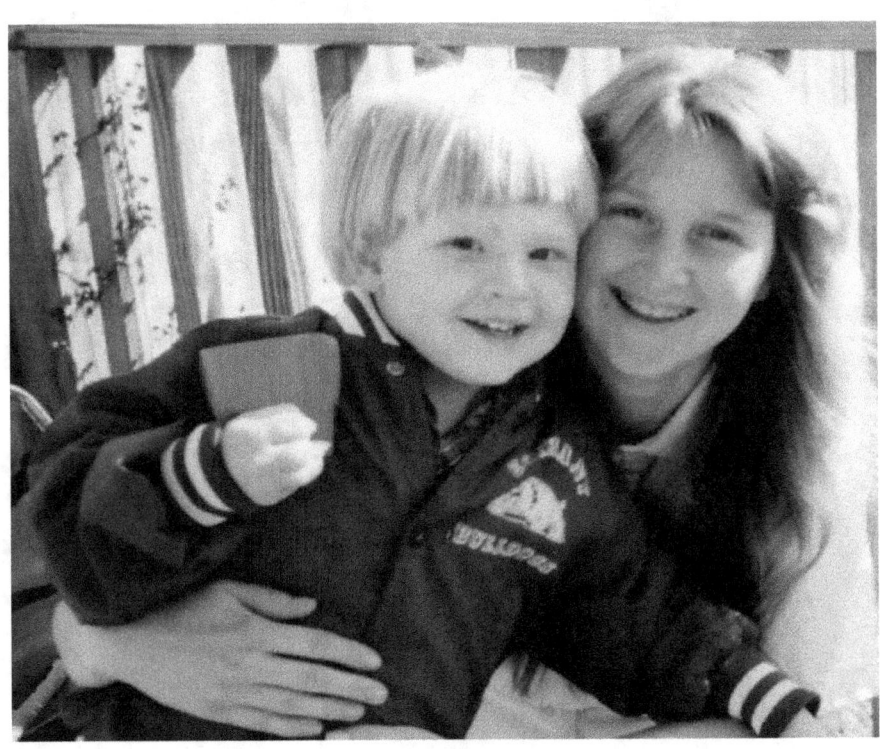

1994

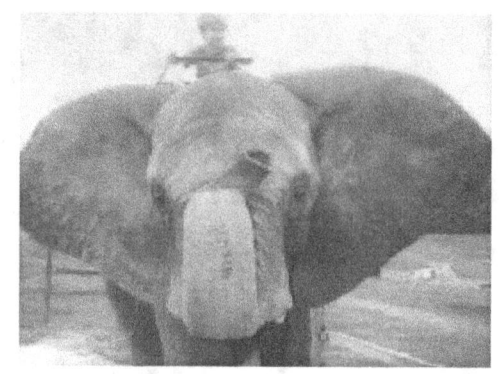

1995

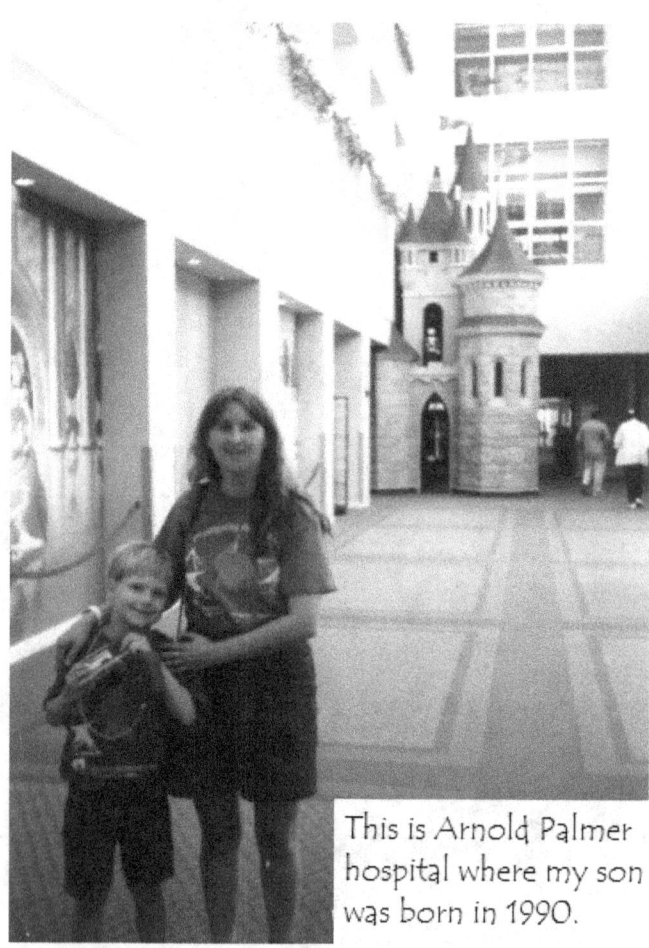

This is Arnold Palmer
hospital where my son
was born in 1990.

1997

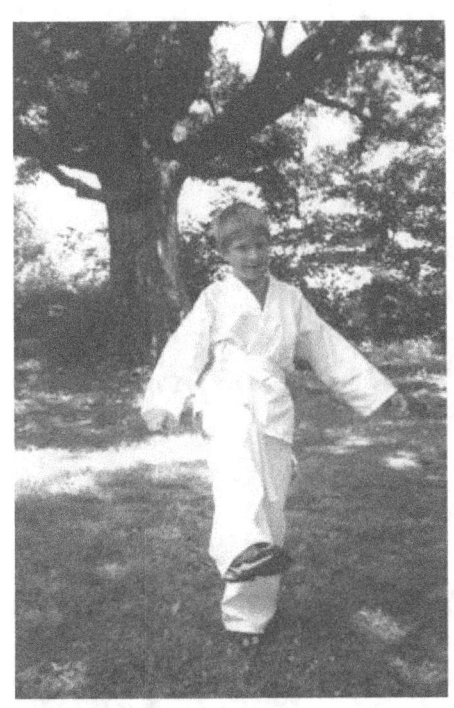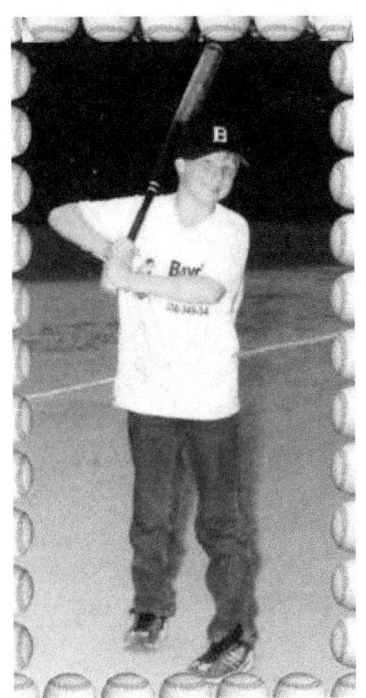

2001

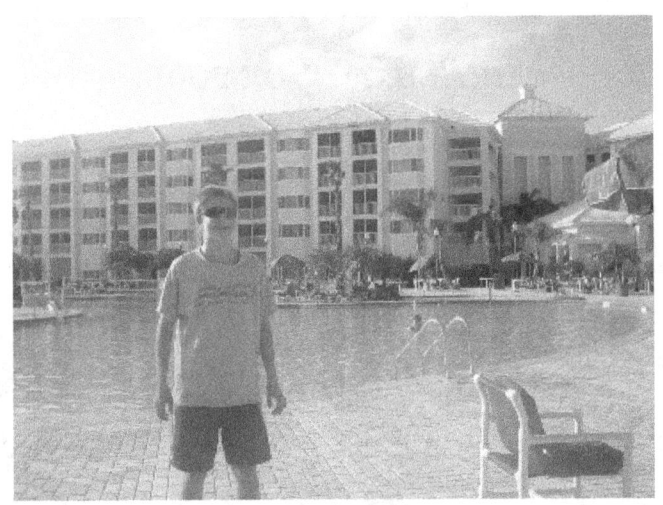

2005

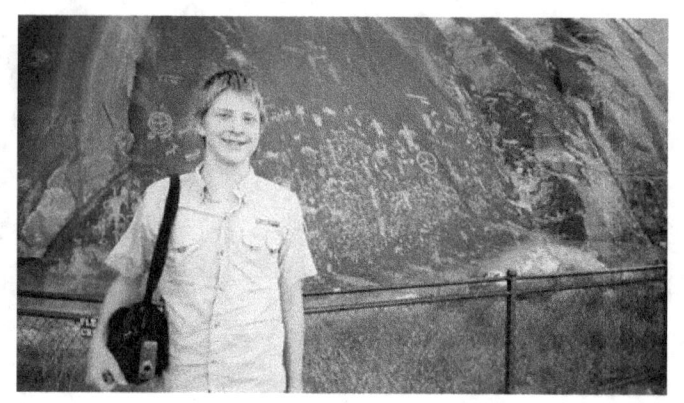

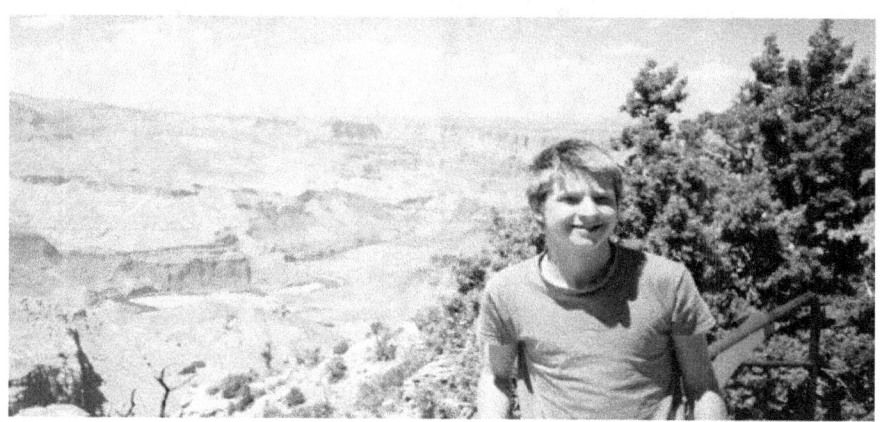

GRAND CANYON 2005

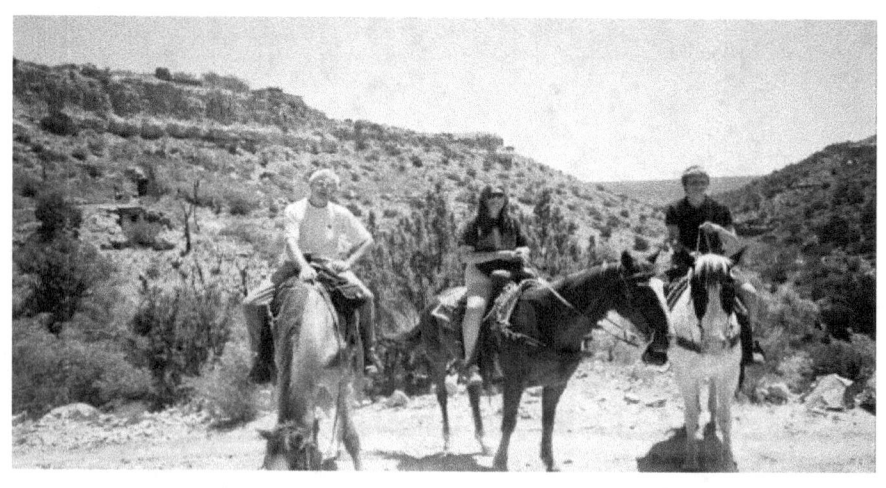

JAMES, ROBERTA & MY          SON 2005

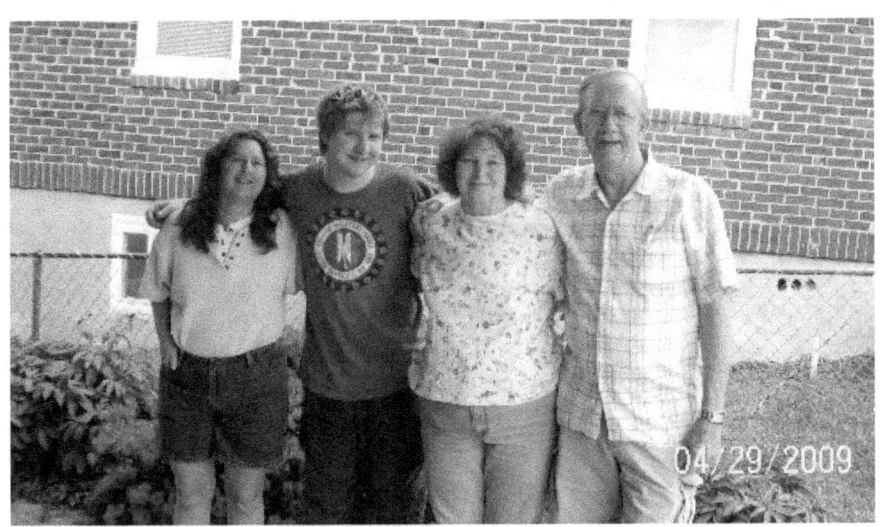

ROBERTA, MY SON, STELLA & KENNY

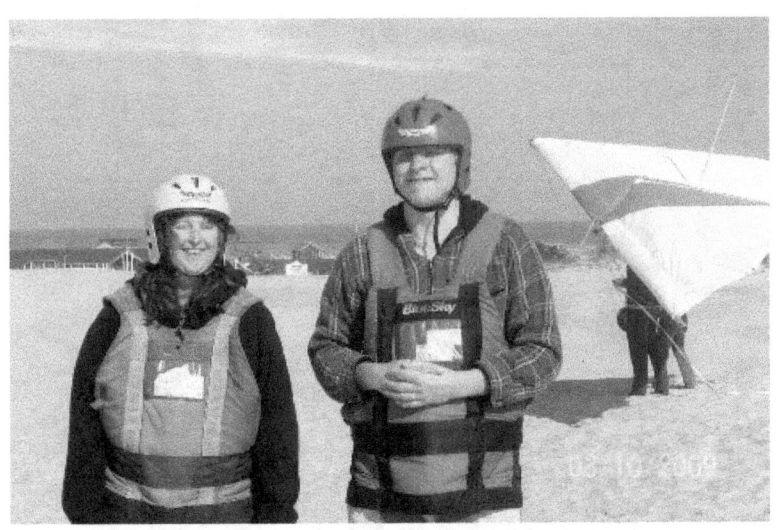

HANG GLIDING 2009

63

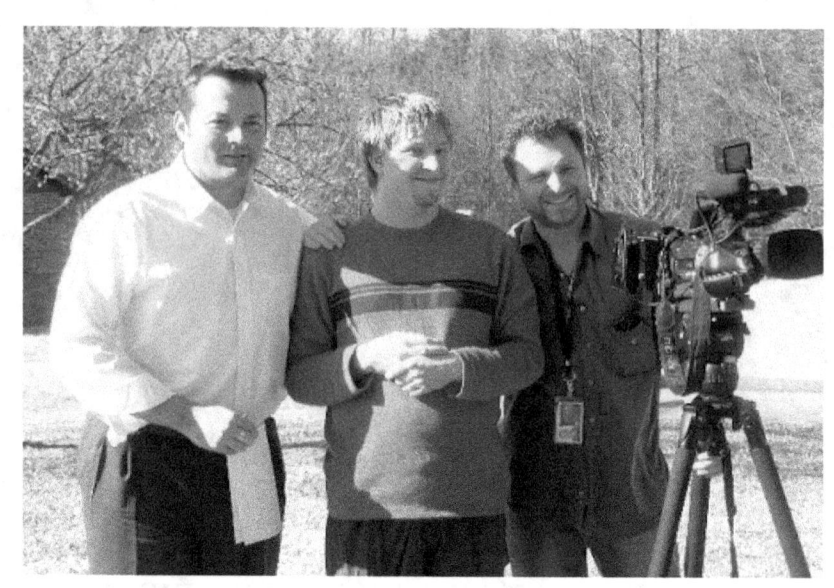

FOX NEWS INTERVIEW 2011

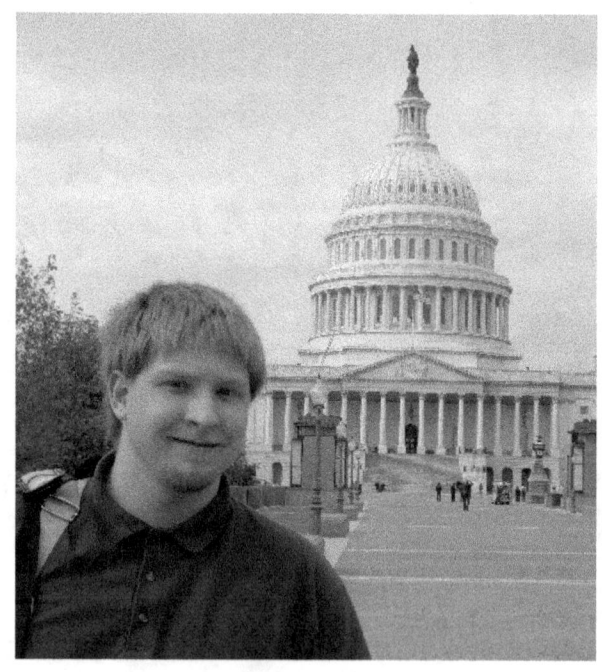

WASHINGTON DC 2011

# KINDERGARTEN AND FINDING A CURE

When my son began kindergarten, I was hopeful that everything would go smoothly, but that hope didn't last very long. On his first day, I heard all kinds of compliments about how polite he was and was amazed that the transition seemed to be going very well, but then the compliments soon faded and became replaced by complaints. He was having really bad tantrums at the school, and the teacher was concerned about how this was affecting the other students. It seemed like they had to call me quite frequently to come and pick him up because of a bad tantrum, and I kept getting notes about his weird behavior. One day, he would just laugh a lot and another day he would be moody and tantrum, and I never knew what was going to happen from day to day.

One day the bus driver informed me that they were going to have to put him in a special harness, because he was having tantrums on the bus and he had ripped out the stuffing in one of the seats. They showed me what the harness looked like and it looked just like the straight jackets that they put on mental patients. After awhile of seeing him put in this thing, I decided that it would be better for me to take him to school everyday. The school paid for my mileage to take him there and pick him up, so I was able to do that even though the school was far away. I just couldn't stand seeing him treated like a mental patient and watching them restrain him everyday in that harness.

Finally everything got to a breaking point, and I was forced to make a decision. The teachers and the principal informed me that I could send him to a rehabilitation hospital for kids with behavior disorders or they were going to have to kick him out of kindergarten. That was their ultimatum and I really had no choice but to admit him into the hospital for an evaluation.

He was admitted to Amos Cottage Rehabilitation Hospital and they started to do all kinds of medical test on him. They did an EEG and found it to be abnormal, and it was interpreted as "abnormal pediatric awake and asleep EEG demonstrating continuous slowing and background slowing." They decided to use a medication to help him with his behavior, they started him on Clonidine. Then they also did a MRI on him, but they didn't find any noticeable abnormalities to his brain.

I was told at a meeting in the hospital that they were having trouble controlling his blood sugars, even with the special diet that they were tailoring to his specific needs. They said that the autism and diabetes work against each other, and that was something that my mom and I had wondered about sometimes. When he had a tantrum, it would make his blood sugar go up and so that made it harder to deal with the diabetes, but also if his blood sugar was high or low, then that would trigger problems with the autistic behaviors. This is precisely what made it so difficult over the years, and I know the combination of these two conditions together created special circumstances that complicated his autistic behaviors.

He stayed in the hospital for about a month, and during this time I decided to move our mobile home onto my parents 5 acres. My mom wanted us to move closer to them because she knew that everything was getting so hard for me, and she wanted to help. Also, the lot rent was going up every year, and we were on a very strict budget, so that was a problem for us.

After being released from the hospital, he returned back to kindergarten, but his behavior never really improved, even with the medication. He would have tantrums after he woke up from his nap, and some of them were really weird. A few times he tried to stomp in the commode and I never really understood why he would even want to do that at all, but he was always doing strange stuff during these episodes. The calls to pick him up early started again, and eventually it ended up in his day being shortened. I started picking him up after lunch and he went for half days the rest of the school year, because most of the tantrums happened after he woke up from his nap.

My son's tantrums had increased in number and intensity, and I was at a loss to explain what would set him off all the time. The things that he got so mad at were so insignificant that they would never upset most people, but to an autistic person just the littlest thing could trigger intense anger and rage. Just going into certain stores seem to trigger him for a tantrum, and we literally couldn't go to Wal-Mart without enduring one. I could never figure out if it was the lights, crowds or the sounds that would set him off, but it always happened. Little things would set him off like sitting in the wrong place, talking to him, smiling at him, putting away toys on the floor, throwing away trash and all kinds of normal everyday things. Back then I always felt like I was walking on egg shells around him, and it was so annoying because I couldn't predict his behavior. I would wake up everyday terrified at having to deal with another tantrum, because I just wanted to live in a peaceful house. I soon became aware that I didn't leave an abusive situation behind when my husband left, so it seemed as if my new situation was like some sick sense of irony. My son would pull hair, hit, kick, throw objects and even bite when he was in a tantrum. All attempts to try to appease him or stop him from this rage was like pouring gas on a fire, and nothing ever worked. I soon found out that he was like a thunderstorm, and I would just have to wait him out and let it run its course to the very end.

When my son was 4 years old, we went to my grandfather's funeral. During the funeral my sister and I had to leave at some point, because we both had small children, so we went outside to let our children run around and play. I was so glad that my son didn't tantrum during the time that the funeral took place, but what happened next at the house was miserable. We all came back to my grandmother's house and started to get ready to eat. My son was putting a whole lot of butter on his biscuit, and I mean he was spreading it all over like it was icing on a cake. My aunt looked funny at me and said something to me about the butter and when I saw what was happening I told him that this was enough and to not put anymore. That was when all hell broke loose; he started screaming at the top of his lungs and ran outside. It was so embarrassing, and I ran after him to try to catch him. He ended up in our car yelling and hitting things while everyone watched in disbelief. My aunt said that she had seen this kind of behavior in the mental hospital where she had worked as a nurse. I know she meant well when she was telling me all of that, but it made me feel weird to know that she was comparing my son to being like mental patients. It was the worst possible moment that I have ever been faced with in my life, and I will never forget that day. I was so embarrassed because this happened in front of so many family members, and it really looked so bad. I could tell that many of them were shocked, because they had never seen anything like this before, but for me this was an everyday thing. They had just got their first real look at the enigma of Autism, and they all looked quite puzzled.

We stayed in a hotel that night after the funeral and instead of getting a good nights rest, we had to endure screaming and crying. It got so bad that we ended up taking my son to the hospital, because we didn't know if there was something physically wrong with him. The doctor examined him and couldn't find anything wrong, so we knew that it was just the autism causing the problems.

Many people don't realize just how difficult it is to visit family or even to attend a social function. I got to the point that I didn't really want to visit any of my family, because I was so afraid that he was going to have another bad tantrum. I can remember that one time our family got together to go up to West Virginia on a trip. I wanted to go, but I knew better, so we never went with the family on that trip. I knew that if we had gone, it would have been hell for my family. This is what it is like to have an autistic child, many times the parents have to sacrifice things that they want to do but know that they can't. Family visits always left me feeling really stressed out because I was afraid during the entire visit that he would tantrum, so many times I tried to eliminate anything that I thought could trigger one and just sat there on edge throughout the entire visit. It wasn't pleasant at all, and I actually started developing headaches and stomach aches before a family visit, because I was totally petrified that he would have an explosive episode.

It was mainly because of the tantrums that I sought a way out of this whole mess, and that also led to some very weird and unforgettable moments. I researched everything I could find about autism and found many things that I could try.

This was a period of time that I tried to find a cure for autism. Many parents will go down this road when they find out about their child, but I think I tried every wacky thing out there that I could afford. Back in the early 90's there wasn't a whole lot of information about what could be the cause of this disability, but I found some possible causes and struck out to test out every one that I could.

I was so thrilled when I found a book about a woman that actually cured her son of autism, just by taking away all dairy products. She found out that her son had a rare allergy to milk that affected his brain and caused him to act autistic. For months, I took away all dairy products, and hoped that I would see a reduction in his tantrums and weird behaviors. At first, my mother and I thought that we noticed some improvements and so I continued, but the tantrums never stopped and I finally realized that it wasn't working and abandoned the diet altogether.

Another thing that I tried actually might have caused more harm then it helped. I had read about a technique called "holding therapy" that I thought might be the answer to all of our problems. This therapy was supposed to address bonding issues between the mother and child, and had helped some autistic children. I felt like maybe we hadn't bonded properly because he was a preemie and was in the neonatal unit for two weeks before going home, so I thought perhaps this might help to correct any issues he might have with me. I found a psychiatrist that was able to do the holding therapy and he was covered by Medicaid. We went to several sessions where we would hold him down, and every time it resulted in a tantrum for the entire session. He was supposed to calm down and give his control over to the doctor, but he never could do that and this therapy never did work. I finally decided not to go back because there was no progress being made, and it was exhausting to hold him down for about an hour while he had his tantrum. Years later my son still talks about how he hated going there and it actually seemed more like abuse to him. I later got his medical files and found out that if the next session had not broke him, that the doctor was going to diagnose him with Bipolar disorder, but we never went back.

I don't know if he has Bipolar or not, but through the years he has been diagnosed with so many things and it is very confusing to me. He has been diagnosed with Pervasive Developmental Disorder, Diabetes Type One, Intermittent Explosive Disorder, ADHD, mild Autism or Asperger's Syndrome, and Duane's Syndrome, as well as other labels that were added and then later dropped.

At one point, we even tried acupuncture to try to help him, but that ended up in a tantrum, so we never went back. I had read that it could help him, and thought that because he gets shots everyday that he would be able to deal with the treatments because it doesn't hurt. In hindsight though, I really don't know what I was thinking about, I guess if someone was coming at me with a bunch of tiny needles to stick in me I would freak out, too.

One thing that I tried that was very popular at the time in trying to cure autism was to find out if he could have any food allergies that could be causing his autistic symptoms. I was able to convince his doctor about taking a blood sample to send to a lab that tested for any kind of a food allergy. I also had him tested for Candida antibodies, which some people were linking to autism, but that test turned out negative. I found out that he was allergic to so many different kinds of foods, but I was willing to cut them all out if it would help him. After showing his diabetic doctor the list of all the allergies to foods, his doctor recommended for us to not eliminate all those foods, because it would end up causing more problems in the long run with his nutrition. I ended up following his doctor's advice.

Another thing that I tried was taking him to a chiropractor for adjustments to his spine and nutritional consultations. He was placed on vitamin supplements and calcium and was taken off of milk and corn products. At first, I thought that I had noticed some improvements, but after awhile it was obvious to me that there was no progress and the tantrums were continuing. Eventually we stopped going and went back to a normal diet again.

Play therapy was a total waste of time, and he did that with no progress either. It was eventually decided by the Psychologist to end the therapy, and I was happy to not have to bring him to therapy anymore.

After trying all of these different things to try to cure the autism or to at least reduce the behavior problems, I would have to say that the vitamins seemed to help the most. Although vitamin therapy never got rid of the autistic behaviors, I did see some small improvements with focusing. During the time that I spent pursuing all of these therapies and treatments, I was so determined to find a cure, but eventually I just accepted that there was nothing that I could do. I think that love and acceptance ultimately are the cure that we all need. When I finally decided to just accept everything and try to focus on his strengths, I found that changing my perspective helped me to see the positive things that I had overlooked. I had been focusing so much attention on trying to find the cure, and spending a lot of time and money for this cause, that I failed to see the whole child before me sometimes. With all the years of school complaints and evaluations that told me everything that was wrong with my child, I felt constantly like I had to fix everything, but in the process you can lose sight of what is really important. Society pressures us into believing that if you don't fit into the majority's perceptions of what is normal, that you need to be medicated or fixed into submission to fit into our world. The pressure is so immense for parents of autistic children to try to get their child to conform, and the parents are conditioned constantly to feel like they are a failure to society. This creates the atmosphere for parents to spend so much of their time and money on anything out there that will give them some hope of a cure, which isn't necessarily wrong, but it takes away our focus on the acceptance of our children as they are. The icon for the Autism Society is a puzzle, because autism puzzles us, but that is ultimately our problem and not theirs. My son has always been an amazing individual and what he has taught me has been very valuable. He has taught me that not everyone has the same perspective on life, but that is alright, some conform to society's norms and some don't. Our need to fix autistic kids is more about ourselves then it is about them, but we do it because we love them and want to see them fit into this society. Perhaps though, our society should also see the positive characteristics of autism, as well. It would help parents tremendously, if they could hear just as much positive observations about their child during evaluations and school meetings, than just hearing about all of the negative stuff.

They say that Einstein might have had autism, because he had the ability to focus on his theories for long periods of time. He was obsessed with his work and persevered on his ideas for hours, which most people are not able to do. All of the major changes with new ideas, technologies, theories and inventions were made by people who dared to be different and not by people who wanted to stay the same. Perhaps autistic people are here to show us that we don't have to all look at this world in the same ways.

What I have learned from watching my son for all of these years is that his perspective isn't always wrong, it is just different. He doesn't like to conform to the clocks control, which most of society does, but that doesn't make him abnormal. He is just more advanced than the rest of us in that he doesn't want to be controlled or enslaved to the clock. Even though this has irked me a lot throughout the years, I secretly admire his freedom to not let time control him. I wish that I wasn't so easily controlled by the clock, but it is our way here, even though it certainly can cause much stress to us all.

Even though I have managed to look at the positive side of autism, it does not mean that I don't still see the negative things. Those things still exist also, and I tried throughout the years to deal with those things that could be life threatening to others and dangerous to himself.

When he was a preschooler and in elementary school, I battled some very dangerous behaviors and it took forever to correct some of them. For instance, my son used to have this bad habit of running around without looking at what was going on around him. Parking lots were a real hazard, and I used to hold his hand very tightly when we had to walk around one. He always seemed to let go of my hand and start running, and so I had to learn to keep a tight grip and keep my full focus on him when there were cars around. For years, I kept talking to him about safety around cars, until finally everything just clicked. With a regular child it doesn't take long to teach them road safety, but for my son it took a very long time.

Another dangerous behavior that he did a couple of times was one of my biggest fears. He used to sometimes start a tantrum in the car, as we were going down the road. A couple of times he actually opened the door, and seemed oblivious to the fact that we were moving. It was the scariest thing, but both times he didn't jump out. When he would start having a blowout tantrum in the car, I would have to pull over on the side of the road and deal with the tantrum until he would calm down enough for me to drive.

I would have to say that my number one safety concern for my son was the tantrums. He had a super strength to him when he had these, and it was not uncommon for him to throw over bookcases, tables and chairs like they didn't weigh anything. I was told by professionals to hold him down during these tantrums, so that he wouldn't hurt himself and others. What the professionals never realized though, is that it was impossible for a single mother to do this all by themselves. Many times after awhile, I would tire out and become exhausted and let go and that is when he would run through the house and throw over things. It was completely impossible for one person to hold down a child for over an hour, while they are having a tantrum. I believe that single parents of autistic children are somewhat set up for failure, as well as parents that are poor, because they can't afford many of the treatments out there or to hire people to help out all the time.

I have to admit here, that I had many meltdowns during this period of my life. Sometimes my mother would come over to my house and help me with the tantrums and I was grateful when she did, but most of the time I was on my own. It was typical, when he was younger, for a tantrum to last over an hour, and those were impossible to deal with always. There were times that I was completely exhausted, and I would just start yelling at my son. Also, I can remember sometimes running out of our house away from him, just so I could have a few moments of peace. Many times through his tantrums, I would start crying uncontrollably and was on the brink of losing my own sanity. Even though it isn't acceptable to yell at your child or run out of the house during a tantrum, when you are totally exhausted and nothing is working, you will do things that you ordinarily would never do. For any single parents of an autistic child, I would have to say don't feel guilty about the meltdowns. You are only human and there are times that you are going to be so exhausted that you won't be thinking properly, that is when you will breakdown. No parent can be a super mom all the time, and so sometimes you're going to make mistakes, but don't feel guilty about your breakdowns. They happen, so accept it when it does and then move on.

I would like to say to all the parents out there, that eventually the tantrums do lessen in number over the years. If my son's tantrums had continued on like that for too many years, then I would have had to place him in an institution, because it is just impossible to deal with that for an entire lifetime. My son is 22 years old, now, and he doesn't have tantrums everyday. He does have small tantrums from time to time, but nothing like he used to go through.

\*\*\*\*\*\*\*\*\*\*\*\*\*\*\*\*\*\*\*\*\*\*\*\*\*\*\*\*\*\*\*\*\*\*\*\*\*\*\*\*\*\*\*\*\*\*\*

## THE PERFECT DAY

I woke up this morning feeling so fine,

I heard the birds and smelled fresh pine.

I went grocery shopping, and they gave away food,

And everyone smiled which showed their good mood.

I looked at the newspaper and they said sickness had gone,

And throughout the whole day I never even felt alone.

Then I picked up my son and he was really feeling great,

And I told him his diabetes was cured as we communicate.

His autism too was gone on this very day,

And we did rejoice and begin to pray.

Everyone we saw was in such a jolly mood,

And life for once seemed to be nothing but good.

People were working together for the first time,

And I saw that there was no more crime.

On that very day not a negative thought came to mind,

Because everyone I met was acting so kind.

The rich and the poor were no longer here,

For we were all equal which made me cheer.

The homeless were welcomed to stay inside,

And then everyone had shelter in which to reside.

No one was going hungry anymore,

And we all knew what life was for.

The air smelled clean with a sweet scent,

And we walked around not caring where we went.

The water in the pond became very clear,

And the animals came all around us, even the deer.

The flowers were brighter than they had ever been,

And the Earth was more beautiful than I had ever seen.

The whole day seemed so perfect to me,

And the angels were visible for all to see.

This was indeed the perfect day,

And I hoped that it would never go away.

I pinched myself to see if I was awake,

But then I woke up and began to shake.

After I had fully awakened, I started to scream,

Then I went back to sleep to relive my dream.

\*\*\*\*\*\*\*\*\*\*\*\*\*\*\*\*\*\*\*\*\*\*\*\*\*\*\*\*\*\*\*\*\*\*\*\*\*\*\*\*\*

# THE SCHOOL YEARS

The next few years I was to endure school problem after school problem, and I never could really enjoy the fact that I had a little free time when he was gone. For most parents, when their child goes to school they can rest easy and be mostly worry free, but for parents of autistic and diabetic children it isn't that way. Everyday, you stay close to the phone or keep your pager on you at all times, and hope that the school doesn't call that day. With my situation, there were always two reasons to call me; either he was having blood sugar problems or behavior problems. I never rested easily when he was at school, because I never knew what was going to happen next. I was on constant call, just like a doctor always has to be available for emergencies, I had to be ready to leave home at a moments notice.

This problem was compounded by the fact that my son still couldn't give his own shots and there was never a full time nurse on duty at his school, so if his blood sugar was up they called me. I would have to go to the school to give him his shot, when this happened. The problem was that with his tantrums and with the autism causing him to get upset quite frequently, well his blood sugar would always get high with all the stress. None of the one-on-one assistants, teacher's aides or any teachers ever did his shots, so I was on call to do the shots when they were needed.

The director of the special education division for the public schools in our county made some changes to accommodate my son's needs. She told my mother on the phone that my son was the most serious case in our county, because he had two health issues. She decided that he needed a one-on-one assistant to help him everyday with his diabetic needs and behavior issues related to the autism, and so they used a program with Mental Health to pay for his assistant. The one-on-one assistant could do the blood test, but none of them ever did any shots, so they would call me when a shot needed to be done.

First grade went like kindergarten and I struggled to go to college in the nursing program and deal with all of the school problems. The calls started again and eventually his days were shortened to half days, and I had to find someone to watch him so I could go to school. A home health care service was able to provide respite care for my son and that helped for a little while, but just before I was to go back to nursing school for my last semester the woman quit coming to watch him. I knew the home health care worker had endured a bad tantrum with him and probably decided that it wasn't worth it for the little bit of money that she made, so I understood why she quit. I knew that it would take awhile to find someone else and then train them, because it had took over a month the last time to find someone to watch him. I made the decision to not continue with the nursing program at this time, because I had no one to watch my son after school and also because of all the problems that he was having.

My mother and I found out about the CAPS program, and I decided to apply for help. The CAPS program helps families that have a child with severe disabilities, so that they won't have to place them in an institution. I managed to get my son on the list, and he was finally approved by the end of 1996. This made it possible for him to get some help, but I soon found out that CAPS would not pay for the therapies that I wanted for him to receive. I wanted to get Applied Behavior Analysis and Auditory Integration therapy, but they said that they couldn't cover those therapies because they were considered experimental and had not been proven to work. During the 1990's though, many families were trying these methods if they could afford them, and were finding that it was helping their children. I was disappointed because I had put in a lot of time and effort into researching about various therapies for autistic children, but was unable to afford them.

CAPS ended up paying for respite care and for client behavior intervention, but ultimately I found the psychologist behavioral intervention methods to be a joke. Instead of reducing tantrums, there seemed to be more tantrums as a result of the different methods tried. He was on CAPS for about two years, but eventually I dropped it because I wasn't really seeing a benefit to keeping these services. The people that worked with him basically had no college training to do what they did, and they just followed the orders of the psychologist.

I can remember one woman that worked with my son during CAPS. She seemed to be doing fine at first, but then I started noticing some weird things. One day she was watching him and so I went out to mow, when all of a sudden I saw her running out of our home. My son was running out after her with a small plastic chair in his hands and he threw it at her. It was so funny to me, because this woman must have weighed about 300 pounds and she was running away from a small kid. I guess she just couldn't hold him down anymore during his tantrum, but that was the way that it was with him because he would have this super strength to him when he was having a tantrum.

Another woman that worked with him before the CAPS program would come out and watch him sometimes, as a part of a respite program, and she was really good with him, but I can remember one time she endured a really bad tantrum. I came home and found her crying uncontrollably in my bathroom. She was completely exhausted and I felt so bad for her, because I knew exactly how that feels.

Another worker that came to our house to watch him under the CAPS program worked real well with my son, but she started getting sick a lot and was unable to work many days and so she ended up quitting. No one ever lasted for very long, and after the CAPS program, I just toughed it out for my self again.

He had a minor surgery when he was 7 years old and when he woke up afterwards he started a tantrum. Many nurses had to restrain him after his surgery and he was never able to calm down fully before leaving the hospital. He was hitting and kicking the nurses, his grandmother and me, while he was screaming very loud. It took 2 nurses to take him to the car and I sat in the back seat with my son while he was having the tantrum. I can remember that his tantrum lasted all the way home, and by the time we had got home I was experiencing another breakdown. I just covered my head and was bent over, so that I could protect myself from his hits, but I just totally went into my own little world. Mom kept trying to talk to me, but I just stayed silent and tried to block out the screaming and everything that was going on. I couldn't help it….I just stopped functioning and stayed in this meditative state for awhile.

Once we got home, my mother and I had to deal with this tantrum for a long time, until finally we were completely exhausted and couldn't deal with it anymore. We called 911, and very shortly an ambulance, as well as many different cars with volunteers showed up in the yard. I was shocked to see so many people had come to help out. For some reason, my son's tantrum started to come to an end after they got there, after hours of this severe tantrum. We decided to take him back to the hospital, but they couldn't find any problems and they attributed everything to being apart of his postoperative pain, which worsened his autistic behaviors. I personally believe that the medicines or anesthesia that they gave him had an adverse effect on him, because his tantrums started to increase in intensity again after he had that surgery.

By the third grade, his tantrums started back up to the intensity that they had once been. Part of that was due to the surgery that he had and part of it was due to his one-on-one assistant having to watch all the kids while the teacher's assistant was out for awhile. My son's classroom was without a teacher's assistant and so the school used his one-on-one assistant for the entire classroom. He wasn't getting someone to help him through his transitions or to help him focus on his work, so his behavior problems started to worsen again. It was almost like it was going back to the days before his assistant, and I could see just how much he needed to have someone there to help him at all times.

I ended up having to admit him to another hospital, so that they could evaluate him and get him some kind of help. He stayed in the hospital for about a week while they evaluated him. He did have some very intense tantrums while he was there, and it took many people to hold him down. They told me that once he started a tantrum that it would escalate and that he was unable to control himself and that there was nothing that they could do beyond that point. They also said that his blood sugar would spike up during these episodes which complicated his diabetes care. They diagnosed him with brittle diabetes, which means that his blood sugars were very hard to control. They also started him on another medication in addition to the Clonidine that he was already taking, and it was called Risperdal.

The school system made the decision to put him in a special education classroom for the rest of the third grade, and they moved him to another school. The teacher was real nice and I felt like she tried really hard to help my son. He still had tantrums, though, even with the two medications, so neither one never really helped him much. I can remember that in this school, they would put him in a closet when he had a tantrum, so that he wouldn't hurt anyone. He continued to go to school for half days at this school.

The fourth and fifth grades went a little better, and he was put more and more into a mainstream class. His classmates were really good towards him and they helped him a lot. He did make some good friends at this school, and I was delighted to see that happen. Even though he had a good one-on-one assistant and a good classroom, there were still some problems. I still had to go to the school a lot to give shots or for other problems, and that kept me from doing other things that I really wanted to be doing. At one point, my mother and I were trying to start our own house cleaning business. We were starting to get some customers and it was nice to have a little extra cash. The problem was that several times we would be cleaning a home and the school would call me. I never knew when this was going to happen, so it made me an unreliable part of the team, and so eventually we just decided to put an end to the house cleaning business.

In 1999, my son had a really bad tantrum at school, which resulted in him being suspended. He hit his one-on-one assistant in the back, and she was injured from this incident. I can remember being called down to the school to meet with his assistant and the principal. It was humiliating. His assistant told me that she could have called the police, because she was assaulted, but thankfully she didn't. I felt really bad about her getting hurt, and was very surprised that this happened.

The whole incident occurred because my son wanted to do his homework, instead of going to music class and it escalated into a tantrum that lasted for 35 minutes. The school system seemed to think that my son could have controlled his behavior, and so they treated him like he was a normal child that had misbehaved. But if it is normal to tantrum because you want to do your homework, rather than go to music class, than most kids would be considered abnormal. I can remember getting upset because I didn't want to do my homework, but I can't imagine getting upset because you can't do your homework. It seemed to me like it was an autistic event, and I disagreed with the decision that the principal had made. I was afraid that now the school would keep suspending him every time he had a tantrum and I knew if that happened, then my son would probably be at home more than at school. My parents and I decided to make a complaint to the North Carolina Department of Public Instruction. They investigated the incident and sent a letter to the school system, so that they could make some changes to try to prevent anymore incidences from occurring again. He was never suspended again after that and my son never injured anyone for the rest of his school years.

The sixth grade was very tough, because the school system moved my son to another school. It just seemed like the cards were stacked against him there, and everyone viewed him in a negative way. My son started to get real negative at this school, and he would spend the entire weekend complaining about all the things that were happening to him there.

I can remember that my son and I read the book "The Diary of Anne Frank" for his school reading program, and we really enjoyed reading that book together and discussing what was going on in her life. I could tell that he comprehended the book, by his questions and our discussions. He took a comprehension test at school one day after he had read the book, and he failed the test, then his English teacher screamed at him. She was upset at him, because he chose to read a book that was above his reading level, and he was reprimanded for his choice. I was very upset when I heard about the days events. He should have been praised for trying to read a higher level book, rather than scolded. I couldn't believe that he failed that test either, because I knew he comprehended that book.

It seems to me that comprehension test don't always show what a person has retained from reading. I just wish that they would have used another approach to measure what he had learned, especially since he has autism. Maybe they should have just asked him about the book, and then he would have told them all that he had learned and remembered about the story. I believe that the educational system has to change. We treat education like it is a one size fits all mentality, but I believe that people learn in many different ways, and teaching should be tailored towards our strengths. My son verbally was explaining to me what was going on in the story, but that knowledge didn't carry over to multiple choice questions, which can sometimes be confusing and misleading.

Another issue at this school was the fact that they did not provide soap or toilet paper in the rest rooms. Each child had to ask the teacher for those items before going to the rest room, and many times there was no soap at all for them to use. My son frequently goes to the rest room when his blood sugar is high and also to wash his hands before a blood test. He was constantly getting frustrated by not having soap, and of course this would set off his autistic behavior, because everything wasn't like it was at home. Without that consistency, it would confuse him, and this experience eventually led to a hand washing routine that he still has to this very day.

There was an incident where he had forgotten to get his eating utensils, and one teacher refused for him to go back and get them. He was ending up having to eat with his hands like an animal, and with all of his classmates watching him. I was very upset about this incident and I made a complaint about this and I told his teacher that she should never have him eating with his hands again.

Eventually, I ended up taking him out of this school and I had him transferred to a charter school in our county.

This worked out fine for awhile in the new school, until his blood sugars started going up everyday and they were calling me to give him his shot. This was about half way through seventh grade, and so I finally decided that it was too much to have to keep going to this school which was 30 minutes away. I made the decision at this time to start home schooling, and we did that all the way up to the tenth grade.

Having him at home everyday was much easier, because I no longer worried about him. If his blood sugar went up, then I could very quickly give him a shot. We started enjoying field trips to many different places, and we both enjoyed the freedom that comes with home school.

I did the best I could to teach my son, and I found out that he was easily distracted, so I had to be brief in our lessons and find entertaining ways to teach him. He has always been into computers, and my son is somewhat of a computer genius, so I used that to teach him quite a lot. Computers always seemed to keep his attention longer, so I would find all of these cool educational websites and it helped tremendously.

My son wanted to learn programming, so we both learned Basic together and I found that I was enjoying learning it with him. We both made some programs during this time and I was so proud of my son for picking it up very quickly. We also both learned some HTML programming for websites, and that was really fun, too.

I just felt like tailoring his learning towards his strengths seem to be the best way to go for him. Home schooling was a challenge though, and I never felt completely comfortable with teaching, however I felt like I did the best that I could possibly do for him. We ended up having school for half a day, and then he was free to work on other projects with his computer.

He ended up learning how to have his own server at 14 years of age and he had his own website that he maintained and promoted. He had more time to focus on his love for computers and I was amazed at all the things that he was learning to do on his own. It is amazing how when we let children have some time to discover things that they like to do, and then they will gladly teach themselves, when it is something that they are interested in doing. I found that my son was learning more with all the extra time that he had, and so home schooling gave him more time to explore all of the possibilities that are out there.

At some point, his doctor switched his injection method from a syringe to an insulin pen, and my son was finally able to learn to do his own shots. He was 14 years old, and I was relieved to not be doing them anymore. The pen made it easier, because you don't have to draw the insulin out of a vial and you just dial up the units. It also had a smaller needle tip to it then a syringe. I still did his night time shot for awhile, though, because my son didn't feel comfortable with drawing out insulin from a vial and using a syringe. Eventually though, when he was 15 years old, his Lantus insulin was switched over to a pen also, and he starting doing that shot, as well. It made me feel good to finally see him become a little more independent with his diabetes care, although I still found that I had to coax him and remind him often to do his shot.

We ended the home schooling when my son was 16 years old, and he decided not to pursue a diploma. I know many people would disagree with that decision, but I am supportive of my son's decision. He knows that he can take a GED course later on if he really wants to pursue that in the future, so that decision is entirely his to make.

My son's school years were challenging, to say the least, and it was a bit of a roller coaster ride through the years. He had many different teachers and assistants that were helpful and very good to him and he had some that weren't, but overall the school system did the best job that they could. My son's circumstances were complicated by the fact that he had two conditions that seemed to work against each other. Obviously, I can't blame his schools for all the problems, because they were financially unable to have a full time nurse. Unfortunately though, this makes it quite difficult on a single parent and I found myself getting frustrated a lot at our situation. I'm sure the teachers didn't like having to call me to give a shot anymore than I hated having to be on call at anytime, but that is just the way that it was.

My son has taught me so much throughout the years, and I am so impressed with him. There is a hidden strength to him that comes from within, and I see how much courage he has in all that he goes through within his life. He has had to work twice as hard to achieve what others have in their life, and I find his life to be an inspiration to me. He deals with high blood sugar, low blood sugar and autistic symptoms constantly in his life, but if you were to see him in a public place you would never know of his struggles. He hides his struggles very well, and he remains upbeat and enthusiastic quite a lot, despite his unfortunate circumstances.

Just to understand what it is like for him, you would have to endure many distractions within your life. What if your communication came from a radio that wasn't tuned in to a good station, and sometimes you got a lot of static and couldn't understand what was being said to you. How would you react to that? I have read some statements by adults with high functioning autism and this is how they describe their lives. They say it is like a radio that is constantly going out and has interference, sometimes the radio station comes in clear and sometimes it doesn't. How would that make you feel if you couldn't always understand what someone was saying to you? Would you get frustrated and possibly have a tantrum? Now, add diabetes to that feeling. Your blood sugar is up and down everyday, and when it is up, your vision gets blurry and when it is down you can't focus or concentrate. Now try to go to school under those conditions and see how well you can do. That is what it was really like for my son, and I am so proud that he did as well as he did. Many years my son made the 'B' honor roll, while enduring all of these characteristics and symptoms. How he did all this, I will never know.

It was a miracle that he did as well as he did all those years. I know God has been watching over him always, and I know that he has given my son a team of angels to watch over him and I am so very grateful.

# AFTER THE AGE OF EIGHTEEN

As my son grew older some problems went away and new problems became increasingly noticeable. Although he still has issues controlling his anger, I have seen him become more tolerable and less explosive than he used to be. He has learned how to calm himself down to prevent tantrums and he very rarely has a tantrum anymore. He still gets angry and sometimes hits furniture, but he is able to regain control very quickly and therefore the situation doesn't spiral out of control anymore. I am very proud of how he has learned to deal with his anger issues.

In his teenage years I noticed he started to add really complex rituals involving hand washing and shower routines. Over the years his routines became increasingly more complex and began to last longer and longer as each year passed. I kept hoping that these routines would eventually go away, but so far they have not. People with autism have additional diagnoses of Attention deficit-hyperactivity disorder (ADHD) and many have Obsessive-compulsive disorder (OCD), as well. According to the A.D.A.M. Medical Encyclopedia, "Obsessive-compulsive disorder is an anxiety disorder in which people have unwanted and repeated thoughts, feelings, ideas, sensations (obsessions), or behaviors that make them feel driven to do something (compulsions)." It is a very debilitating disorder which takes over every facet of the person's life.

There are times that I observe my own life and I can't believe how strange my world has been compared to the average family. Every time we get ready to go to a doctor's visit or to go anywhere it has almost become an all day event. If we go somewhere in the morning, then I have to get him up very early in the pre-dawn hours, since he has all of these routines that take hours to perform. When it first began it would take an hour for him to go through his shower routine and to get ready. As of writing this book it currently takes about 4 hours for him to get ready to go anywhere. Yes, 4 hours! People have no idea how much time people with OCD spend on just repeating the same procedure over and over again. It is almost painful to watch what he does each time. He literally washes his hands and arms so much that they are red and sometimes the skin peels and bleeds. Doctors keep prescribing various ointments, lotions and creams to help with his ever growing skin problems, but unless my son stops with these elaborate hand washing routines I don't see them doing any good.

His normal shower routine is for him to lay out his clothes on a towel in the bathroom. He goes into the bathroom and I won't hear water running for quite sometime. He starts talking to himself and I have no idea what he does for like 30 minutes to an hour before he actually turns on the shower. For the next hour he will take his shower, and then it could be another 30 minutes to an hour before he leaves the bathroom. You would be shocked at how much our water bill has ballooned up to over the years and how much we spend on soap. The bathroom is always a wreck after he is done, there are towels lying on the floor everywhere and some of them are completely soaked. The floor will have water all over the place and the toilet is usually un-flushed with a pile of toilet paper inside. Sometimes I would have to use a plunger just to get the          commode to flush.

Once he actually leaves the bathroom, he proceeds to the kitchen where he then does an elaborate hand washing routine for 20 to 30 minutes. He also washes his hair at the sink with soap and water and not shampoo anymore. He gets suds all over his hair and his face and he looks so funny that sometimes I want to laugh, but refrain from doing so. Once he has completed his routine, then he will get his shirt, socks and shoes ready. The next routine is for him to wash his pants, while he is wearing them, even though they were already washed in a washing machine. By washing his pants, I mean he soaks them down with water, and this gets water and soapy suds all over the kitchen floor. This makes it completely difficult to take him anywhere in the wintertime due to the fact that he is soaking wet after he is done. His final routine is when he washes the bottom of his shoes before putting them on. There is no apparent reason that I know of for why he does all of these routines, but it seems to help him with the transition of leaving the house.

People would be shocked to see the things that I have seen over the years. My son talks to himself quite a lot and he often carries on conversations with himself throughout the day. He talks to himself sometimes while he is on his computer, most of the time when he washes his hands and arms and most of the time when he takes a shower. It is always interesting to watch someone's reaction that hears him for the first time talking to him self. Usually, I will get the question "Who is he talking to?" "No one", I would reply, and then I would get to see a very perplexed look on their face. It was a normal thing for me to hear everyday, but to other people it was a very strange thing to experience. We all have conversations with ourselves, so really this is quite normal, but the only difference is we use our inside voices, whereas my son would verbally say every thought that came into his mind. It was actually quite fascinating sometimes to just listen to his elaborate conversations with himself. Many times he would go through an entire daydream sequence of expressing a fantasy storyline that he was experiencing in his mind. Sometimes he was saving the world and other times he was falling in love with a character he met in his dream world. With most people you sometimes wonder what is going on inside their head, but with my son everyone knows his every thought at times.

My son decided to start a website at one point, and so I agreed to pay a monthly fee for a website server with good bandwidth. I was astonished to see what he did with his alternative news website over the years. He put together a very professional looking website with a scrolling news panel of pictures and text. He wrote his own articles and would take very professional looking photos that he also used on his website. When we went out west on a trip with my mom and step dad my son had made little paper cards on the computer about his website and so he handed them out and left them at various places around the country. He was a genius at knowing how to promote his website and I watched how his followers grew over the years. He also successfully established a You Tube channel and had many followers on there, as well. At one point, he started to promote his website on Facebook and that brought even more people to his website. He had thousands of people going to his website everyday. It was simply amazing to watch him!

But for every upside of autism there is a downside, and I quickly learned that having a very successful website on alternative news will get the person noticed in the most unfavorable ways. His website was constantly being attacked by hackers and so that became a major battle at some points, because my son had to keep saving backups of his website for restoring purposes. There were many times that he had to keep dealing with these hacker attacks and it made his website a headache at times for him to manage. He ran the whole thing by himself, so he learned everything he could about how to make websites, how to research and write articles, as well as how to promote his website. I learned quite a lot just watching him do all of those things.

Our next greatest battle was so hard to get through and it actually ended up leading to more health issues in the process. My son posted a picture that he got on another website and he put a link back to the website which is the acceptable way to share information on the web. This picture was of a man being patted down by a TSA agent in the airport. This particular photo had gone viral and it was all over the World Wide Web and so anyone that looked up information on Google about the TSA would have seen this photo under the images tab. So many websites were reposting this photo over and over again. He was sued for copyright infringement by a company called Righthaven, and it was a very devastating experience for us. We first heard about the lawsuit from a reporter in Las Vegas before my son was served the papers. The lawyer called us up and tried to get us to pay a settlement of $6,000, but my son and I refused the offer for a settlement. We told the lawyer that we didn't have that kind of money and that my son was living off of SSI disability for autism and brittle diabetes. The lawyer was very cold and threatened to take money out of his SSI each month. I told him that we were going to go to the media with what they were doing to my son and he told us to go ahead and do that if we want. I was so proud of my son, because he pursued every way he could to get his story out to the media. He called reporters at many different newspapers to try to get an interview. There were many newspapers that did interview him and so Righthaven started to get a lot of bad publicity. My son did all of this by himself and it was quite interesting for me to watch him calling all of these reporters and doing many interviews.

At this time, my son was 20 years old and we had started to visit his dad a couple of times. His dad arranged for him to be interviewed by 2 local TV stations in our area. We were ecstatic about the interviews and happy to see that his dad finally did something to help his son. My son did an amazingly wonderful job on both interviews. If I had done the interview, I would have been really nervous and I'm sure I would have made a lot of mistakes, but he was really calm and he answered every question eloquently. I was so proud of him. He learned how to work the public relations with the media and became a PR nightmare for Righthaven. The most interesting interview that my son did was for the New York Times, and this particular article has been read by people all over the world. Righthaven kept trying to make settlements where they were trying to take away his rights to ever talk about this lawsuit or Righthaven forever, but we did not settle with them.

My son started to have really bad seizures during the time period of this lawsuit. Some were so bad that it would take over an hour for his blood sugar to get back to normal. This was such a very depressing time for me, because I was dealing with seizures day and night and I never knew what to expect. He was also having a lot of falls and some minor injuries with these severe insulin reactions and the seizures, but I tried to prevent falls whenever I could. The problem was that he had started to gain so much weight after he became an adult, so it became increasingly harder to help him when he was stumbling around low. I couldn't help him get up off the floor when he fell and so many times I was treating these insulin reactions on the floor, which wasn't the most comfortable thing to do. There was one night that I woke up because I heard a loud thud noise in the middle of the night and my son was on the floor downstairs having a full blown seizure. Many objects had been knocked over including his laptop computer, and so I struggled to clear out the mess and give him icing to bring up his blood sugar. So many times I wonder why he is still alive after seeing how quickly he can have a seizure day or night, but somehow I always catch these and give him the icing that he so desperately needs. There have been times that I have awakened in the middle of the night and my first thought is to check my son's blood sugar and when I do, it is always low. I've always had the feeling that his Angels wake me up to help him and I feel very grateful and blessed to be given their special help anytime day or night.

I have a friend named Gary A. David, who is a professional writer and has recently been interviewed by the History Channel for many different programs. He has written the book "The Orion Zone" about a discovery that he found of a star map that was formed from Native American villages in Arizona. He also has an adult daughter with autism, and so he personally understands about the plight of autism on young adults. He suggested that we get in contact with a local newspaper in Colorado that he knew about, so my son did get in contact with them and they interviewed him over the phone. It was because of this particular interview with Westword Newspaper that my son got a pro bono lawyer to represent him in this lawsuit. I was grateful for Gary's tip to contact this newspaper, because this led to my son getting the legal help that he so desperately needed.

A lawyer named David Kerr read the article in the Westword Newspaper and decided that he wanted to help my son. He worked for a law firm named Santangelo Law Offices, and so he approached his boss about possibly representing my son for free on this particular case and his boss agreed to do so. My son and I were very grateful to receive this legal help. I had already responded to the legal papers that my son was served with and not knowing anything about law I did it all wrong. Thankfully, Mr. Kerr read through what I had submitted to the court and he saw that I had not responded correctly, so he wrote to the court to let them know that my son now had a lawyer and that we needed an extension. The judge granted the extension and the law firm took over from there, and it was such a weight off of our shoulders because we knew we were in good hands and that everything was going to be okay. It took a few months but eventually with all of the bad press that Righthaven had received, and due to the fact that my son now had a lawyer, of course, Righthaven finally backed down and dismissed the lawsuit. Our nightmare had finally come to an end and we never had to pay any money to Righthaven.

The seizures continued however and so I was desperate to get some kind of help. I got video of one of my son's more unusual seizures and insulin reaction and I took it to his doctor.  The doctor looked at the video and he referred me to a neurologist, so I took my son to the appointment and they did an EEG test to look at how his brain was functioning.  The test came back abnormal, and the neurologist said that he didn't feel comfortable prescribing medicine for the seizures since they have so many side effects.  I was happy with that decision to not put him on medication, but at the same time this didn't solve the problem.  I had been talking to my son about reducing his insulin to see if that would help, but he is stubborn and he kept refusing to reduce his insulin amount.  Finally, though at one point, I was able to get him to start reducing his long acting insulin of Lantus, and I did notice a reduction in seizures and the few that he continued having weren't as bad and didn't last as long.  At least, we were starting to conquer some of his health issues and I was starting to feel more secure in my job of taking care of him.

My son was really getting into making videos for his You Tube channel and writing articles for his very successful website.  He was making friends and he was doing interviews for his website and You Tube channel, which were increasingly getting lots of views.  As I wrote before, he was getting thousands of hits a day on his website, and he had to temporarily take it down during the lawsuit, but afterwards he was able to put it back up again.  He also had a lot of followers on Facebook, as well as on You Tube, so I was very amazed at what all he was creating for himself.  He started really researching about politics and law, which propelled him to write very interesting articles on many different topics.  There were several of his articles being posted to even bigger websites, such as Alex Jones' website called Prison Planet.

If my son had not had autism, diabetes and seizures, I could really see where he may have been a lawyer or a politician. He might have also been a business man too. He is very intelligent, and he also has this ability to know how to promote and market his ideas, as well as the fact that he is also quite creative. Even with all of the obstacles that he has had to face in his daily life, he managed to do things that other people might only have dreamed of doing in their life. Despite his mild autism, he is outgoing and friendly to everyone he meets, and despite the diabetes and seizures he still manages to do many things that he wants to accomplish without the fear or worry over his health. I am constantly amazed at what he has been able to do in his life despite all of the obstacles placed before him.

He has interviewed many people for his website and You Tube videos and some of these people are real well known or famous. He has interviewed Orly Taitz (lawyer), Virgil Goode (Presidential candidate 2012), Jim Tucker (author & reporter), Eldon Crisman (scientist), (author & scientist), Pastor James David Manning, Tea Party Founder Dale Robertson, Preston Nichols (author & scientist) and many more people. This is quite impressive considering his disability and chronic illness!

One day he started talking to me about making a documentary and he started to plan everything that he wanted to do. I was impressed with how he made this goal for himself and then I got to watch how he planned out every detail and worked towards fulfilling his dream of making his own documentary. He did everything by himself, which is the way he worked on his website, as well. When we went to Washington D.C., he kept filming sequences for the video and he would go up to strangers and ask them questions about the government. This is something that I could never do and I don't have a diagnosis of autism, but I am quite shy, so I was very impressed with how he had the courage to do that with total strangers.

After he finished his documentary, I watched the whole thing and was so amazed at how professional it looked with all of the various special effects that he used. I must say that I also learned a lot from him about using special effects in my own videos. He is very talented as a filmmaker, too, and I think that whatever goal he sets for himself he can achieve it when he really tries.

My parents and I spent a month trying to get help for him at one point during a recent crisis and we could not find any kind of immediate help. It has been months since I put my son on the list for group homes and I still have not heard any word from them, and I've seen on the internet where it could be years for him to get into a group home.

My son is now 22 years old and my life and his has changed significantly last year when we decided to move into our own apartments. My parents offered for me to move into some apartments that they bought a few years ago and I should have, but for some reason I didn't want to move back then. Recently however, we did make the decision to move to Virginia and we love living here. My son moved into a basement apartment and I moved into the upstairs apartment, which isn't that far from him, so I can still check up on him and test his blood sugar when he is sleeping. This move has worked out very well for us, and it is wonderful for both of us to have our own place now, yet still be      close to one another.

I found out about a Medicaid program that would be beneficial for my son, so I enrolled him in that program at social services. They sent out two people to do the evaluation and they put me in contact with a local home health care. The woman that owned the home health care came out and offered me the job to be a care provider for my son, so I quickly accepted. I could not be a paid caretaker before because we were living in the same house, but now that my son has his own apartment it is acceptable. I've been doing the job for free since he turned 18 years old, so it was a surprise for me to see that I can now get a paycheck. The home health care could have hired anyone to do this job, but since I already have 22 years experience it makes perfect since to let a family member or parent be the caregiver. This has opened a new door for me and it gives me the opportunity to finally get some money, pay into social security and to now have something to put on my resume. I am so excited to now have a job and to finally have a little more money to buy the things I need and to be able to do more now.

I've been writing books for a few years now and putting them online, as well as writing poems that I have put on websites. I was never able to publish any of them, because my son and I lived in the same household and it would have affected his SSI and his Medicaid. I felt not only tethered to my son over his health care, but I felt held back financially, as well. I was not able to make any money or my son could possibly lose his Medicaid. This was a source of worry over the years, because his medicines and supplies are around a thousand dollars a month and that doesn't include doctor's visits or hospitals. I would have liked to find a way to work from home and watch him at the same time, but I knew he could possibly lose his Medicaid and with his diabetes and seizures I was afraid to lose his good medical care. Once our finances became separate from living in our own apartments, I was finally able to make money without affecting his health care. This has freed me to actually think about my own finances again without worrying about his medical expenses. I am finally free to explore financial opportunities that were not an option before. I submitted one of my books to a self publishing company that prints on demand for any orders that I get, and so I can finally make some money from one of my books after all of these years. At the same time, I am also getting paid for 4 hours a day to care for my son and to deal with the seizures and insulin reactions. This job will also benefit him because now I can do more for him then I could before, since I have more money for what he wants or needs. We always had to pinch pennies before, but now I don't have to be on that tough budget anymore, so with this job comes more freedom and less worrying over finances. My life has changed so much in these last few months and I am very grateful, as I feel blessed to be there for my son and yet to be able to have more freedom within my own life again. I don't mind all the years that I sacrificed for him, because I wanted to be there for him, but now it feels good to be able to do some things just for me again.

Both diabetes and autism are on the increase around the world right now, and it is debatable at this time as to what is causing the increase. It is shocking to think that in our modern times of having the best health care than the world has ever known that we are also seeing more sickness than ever before, as well. When my son was first diagnosed with autism it was affecting 1 in 10,000 but now it is affecting 1 in every 88 children. That is a really big increase over the last two decades, and so many more people will be affected by the things that my son and I have experienced in the last 22 years. One of the reasons that I wanted to write this book was to be able to let young parents know that they are not alone in what they are experiencing. Back when I was raising my son up, I mostly felt all alone, because no one in my family had children with autism, so there was no one that I could talk to about these things that would understand. My world was so much different than other people's realities and so I couldn't relate to them and they couldn't relate to my life. This alienated me from the world in so many ways and I no longer fit into the norm. It was frustrating to deal with so many challenges over the years and with nothing there to help me. Everything that I knew of parenting involved my normal middle class upbringing with two parents, and so I couldn't really do things the way that my parents did when they raised me. I had to be both the mom and the dad to my son and I had to do more controlling with strict supervision for my son than my parents did for me, because of his very brittle diabetes and the autism. I couldn't let my son just go play with the other kids in the neighborhood all day, because of his health I had to watch him closely. I was always worried day and night that something could happen to him when I'm not there, and now that he is grown nothing has changed, because I still worry. I have always been his only caretaker and so everything falls on me to keep a vigilant watch over him at all times. I have to check blood sugars when he is sleeping and be there to assist him at all times whether it is day or night. It would be an impossible job if I felt like I didn't have any help from above. It has been mostly my faith in God and his team that helps me to feel like I can be there for him when he needs me. I rely on this spiritual help that I have got more than anything else to help me to take care of him. If I ever get a strong feeling or urge to check on my son whether it is daytime or in the middle of the night, I always trust in that guidance or God given intuition that comes from within. It is always this guidance that has got me through my job as a parent and that gets me through each and every day too. Without my faith in God, I would have been lost a long time ago and would have never been able to take care of my son.

Raising a child with diabetes, seizures and autism as a single parent has been the most challenging job that I have ever done in my life. With other jobs, I got recognition, money and a schedule, but with this job I didn't get those kinds of rewards. I was paid in love and I was never fully recognized for all that I did, but usually for all that I didn't do or for my many mistakes. I have no idea what a work schedule is because my work schedule is to be there for him at anytime...... day or night. I've saved his life more times than I can ever remember, and yet I would like to forget. No parent should ever have to see their child have a seizure or be forced into giving shots everyday to their child for 14 years and yet I was, but despite having to endure this situation as nightmarish as it could be, we have gotten through it just fine.

When I look back at everything we have been through, I can't help but think how could we have possibly got through all of this and yet have maintained our sanity. When my son was about 14 or 15 years old we went whitewater rafting for the first time. I can remember going in between big boulders and over small waterfalls while zig zagging our way through a rocky maze within the roaring current of the river. I can remember looking back one time and seeing all of the boulders that had been in our path and I wondered how the heck we got through. This is what it was like as a single parent raising my son, I look back now and I wonder how on Earth we got through all those obstacles that were placed in our way. When we were whitewater rafting, we had a guide telling us which way to paddle and guiding our every move on the course of the river. When I was raising my son, I also had guides telling me what to do when I was met with all of these obstacles, and became reliant on listening to my guides in everything that I did. My guides are God, Christ, the Holy Spirit and the Angels, and I have also learned to trust my inner instincts or my God given intuition to guide me in my endeavors, as well. My advice to every parent that is going through what I have gone through is to learn to trust your intuition and let God and his teams guide you along your path. You will be amazed at all the obstacles that you will get through together and someday you will look back on your life and see the beauty in what all you have learned.

My son has done some amazing things and I have enjoyed watching his many talents unfold. He is very ambitious and he has tried so very hard to make something wonderful of his life, despite the many obstacles that have been placed in his way over and over again. Anyone can accomplish many things in their life when they have been given the best of health, no disabilities and have been raised with a lot of money or in a two parent family, but my son had none of those things and yet he has accomplished so many different things in his life so far. He didn't have the advantages that most

children in America have had, but he still persisted to try
new things and to make many goals for himself that he
did accomplish despite the cards constantly being stacked
against him. I am proud of all of his accomplishments
big and small, and I feel that there is nothing that my son
can't do if he sets his mind to a certain task. His autism,
seizures and diabetes do not define him; they are just
merely his obstacles. He lives with these obstacles
everyday, but he doesn't let them get in his way of doing
what he wants to do and for that he is to be commended.

✱✱✱✱✱✱✱✱✱✱✱✱✱✱✱✱✱✱✱✱✱✱✱✱✱✱✱✱✱✱✱✱✱✱✱✱✱✱✱

## The Lawsuit

They sue my son out of greed,
well, they had better take heed.
Taking from the disabled and poor,
will never make your company grandeur.
I've never talked to a lawyer so cold,
and one so uncompassionate and bold.
Two phone calls made me feel so down,
lost and harassed, and left me with a frown.
Big corporations don't give a damn,
and buying copyrights to sue is a scam.
It figures your headquarters is in sin city,
a gamblers paradise, what a pity.
Attacking people for sharing the news,
and harassing them with extortion abuse.
Preying on the innocent for cash,
talking in a manner that is brash.
Harassing someone with autism is cold,
while trying to take his money and scold.

For money: they lie, harass, cheat and sue,
and they don't care what they put him through.
Stress can make his blood sugar so high,
while they call and harass and pry.
Preying on the poor and the sick,
using old newspaper articles is their trick.
Beware of copyright infringement scams,
these wolves are going after the lambs.

**About the author:**

Roberta Hill is a home health care worker, writer and researcher. She has her own You Tube channel where she makes videos on the RH negative blood type, physics, astronomy, Coral Castle, poetry, animation, sacred geometry and various other subjects. Her channel is called TheStarchild2009. She has written numerous online research books and poetry.

www.ingramcontent.com/pod-product-compliance
Lightning Source LLC
Chambersburg PA
CBHW070539290526
45790CB00002B/570